MW00831649

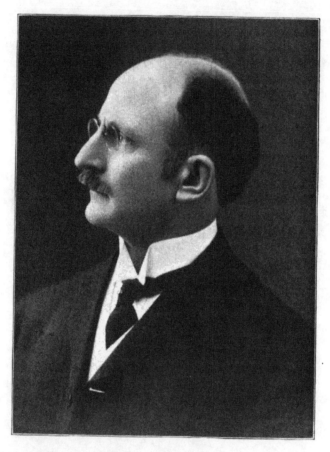

Yours for health

E. J. Bartholomew —

Osteopath & Oculist

MAN, WOMAN KNOW THYSELF!

AN ILLUSTRATED TREATISE ON PRACTICAL PSYCHOL-
OGY FOR BOTH THE MEDICAL PROFESSION
AND THE LAITY

A PRACTICAL, SCIENTIFIC EXPLANATION OF THE
EFFECT OF THOUGHT—THE MYSTERIOUS
FORCE WHICH DETERMINES ONE'S
CONDITION IN THE PRESENT
AS WELL AS THE FUTURE
LIFE

BY

DR. ELMER JEFFERSON BARTHOLOMEW

6
W
1908
2

CONTENTS.

PREFACE.

Know thyself: These words, generally speaking, have little significance for the average being.

The farmer knows all the peculiarities and fine points of his horses, cattle, sheep and swine; he goes into minute detail regarding their breeding and the care they require; the successful business man masters all the intricacies and requirements of his trade; the architect devotes great thought to the plans for the building to be constructed; the housewife acquires, eagerly, every bit of knowledge conducive to the good government of her domain, but neither the farmer, business man, architect nor housewife takes sufficient interest in Self or endeavors to gain knowledge of that which should concern him most—his own body!

He has but a superficial knowledge, if any, of its parts—of the relation of its parts to each other and to that Mysterious Force governing them.

Mankind's principal study should be man! Being absorbed in professional enterprise, he fails to consider that the accumulation of his Cash Bank

15

Account and its maintenance depends absolutely upon his Vital Bank Account.

Therefore, I will endeavor to demonstrate to the medical profession, as well as the laity, how diseased conditions are produced, how avoided; and how health may be maintained or restored, thus insuring the Vital Bank Account and in turn the Cash Bank Account.

The physician often absolutely disregards the relation of mind to the body and endeavors to remove the evident disability. of a patient without tracing it back to first principles.

When treating disease the medical profession should never lose sight of the fact, which has generally been the case heretofore, that the energy which runs the human machine (the body) is nerve force; that this nerve force is generated in the brain and conveyed therefrom by the nerves to all parts of the body, supplying them with energy, life, vitality; that the mind is the engineer governing the amount of nerve force generated in and radiated from the brain; that the human machine is similar to all others; that all machines are built for some special service, and that there are only two ways by which they can be rendered unserviceable: by a mechanical defect (such as a slipped cog or broken axle) or by handicapping the engine that generates the force or energy necessary to run it.

To simplify these remarks, explanations by pictures and comparisons will be used to show that disease is an effect, produced by a cause; that the cause must be eliminated to remove the effect; that both mental tension and mechanical pressure produce disease, with mental causes largely in the majority.

If there are any exceptions to the above rule it is with children who appear to have a toxic or poisonous substance in the system which it is necessary to eradicate, and is generally eliminated by diseases diagnosed as measles, mumps, whooping cough, etc., but there is a doubt in my mind that children would have even these diseases, were their circulation not impeded by colds and other abnormal conditions of the nervous system.

As to the force which runs the human machine (the body), I first invite your attention to a few paragraphs regarding the mind, its origin, function and development—also to thought, from whence it comes, for what purpose and its effects.

THE AUTHOR.

"Were I so tall to reach the pole,
  Or grasp the ocean in my span,
I must be measured by my soul,
    The mind's the standard of the man."
                              —*Watts.*

MIND, ORIGIN AND DEVELOPMENT.

In all ages of man, the paramount wonder or subject for discussion has been the mind or the soul.

The mind or soul represents the measure of thought (energy, intelligence, life, electricity, if you so wish to call it) that we possess, that is, the amount we have "stored away." By this, we mean that our mind represents the amount we possess of the All-pervading Intelligence—the All-pervading Energy—the All-pervading Mind, Wisdom or Force that is in everything, surrounds everything, of which everything is made, is ever present and known as God.

The quality of our mind, or rather our marked traits of character, were "handed down" to us through our mother's mind (as a channel) during our pre-natal existence. Our post-natal development has been influenced largely by the pre-natal influences, in conjunction with environment, reading, observing, communing and placing our mind in tune with the Infinite Mind, of which our mind is part.

21

ONE'S MIND LIKE A STORAGE BATTERY.

Each individual mind has attained its present development by absorbing or acquiring intelligence by attracting it—the mind has been placed in a condition to receive intelligence as one would arrange a storage battery for re-charging. A storage battery is charged by attaching it to that from which it receives or absorbs electricity (strength, vitality, life, energy).

The battery represents the amount of electricity (energy, life, intelligence) that it has absorbed, so the mind represents the measure of thought (the amount of the All-prevading, Infinite Intelligence, life, force or energy) that it has attracted and retained.

The force in the storage battery (called electricity), when released and conveyed through the proper channels, will run your automobile. In like manner will the force (thought), of which the human storage battery (the mind) consists, operate the human machine (the body) when released and properly transmitted through the nervous system.

All forces (like thought or nerve force, electricity, steam, etc.) are the same in substance, generated under different conditions, but derived from the one, All-pervading Force, God, thus the soul or mind (from which thought issues) must

22

be of God, as a drop of water is part of the ocean.

The quality of mind determines the status of life, for the mind is the gate-keeper or guardian of the soul, and conscience is one of its divine attributes.

When conscience is troubled the mind is troubled. When one experiences a spiritual or soulful change the condition of mind is changed. A change of heart, an expression frequently used, is also a change of the state of mind.

Mind can not deceive that of which it is a part; neither should one mind try to deceive another, both being derived from the same source and part of the same Infinite Mind.

THE BODY AND FIVE SENSES SERVANTS OF THE MIND.

The mind uses the brain as a key-board to transmit nerve force (brain fluid, thought or electricity) through the nerves (live wires) to the different muscles of the body, causing them to contract and approximate the bones to which they are attached, resulting in speech or action.

Our thoughts precede our words and actions, therefore our present condition in life is the result of our thoughts. Our future condition in this life and the future life will depend entirely upon our thoughts.

The mind or soul is the tenant of the human dwelling, and all the functions of the body (including the five senses) are servants of the mind.

28

The mind commands these servants that it may prosecute its work or wishes, and thereby progress and develop.

Thought precedes words and actions! Then every creature capable of uttering a sound or moving must possess a mind or soul, and the accompanying thought consistent with its mental development.

THE IMPORTANCE OF BODY AND MIND TO EACH OTHER.

Human thought, if not vented in speech or action becomes inert, thus hindering mental development. This fact, alone, should convince the reader of the importance of body to mind or soul; for, if one wishes to clothe thoughts in words, how possible without the vocal organs (lips, teeth, tongue, palate and vocal cords)? Or, if one's thoughts are such as would precede action, how can action be produced without the servants of the mind (the muscles, body, arms, fingers, legs, feet, etc.)?

God's slogan is "Eternal Progression," brought about by the advancement of man's mind or soul. It is impossible for man, during this life, to attain mental perfection, else he would not require a body of flesh and blood during this existence.

The theologian tells us, that if the earthly life be encompassed by the creed which he represents, the future existence will be in the spirit and not in the flesh. How absurd! God does not intend that man, either in this or in his infinite number of future lives, shall reach the state of mental perfection, which if attained, would enable him to cope with God's wisdom. Just as long as the immortal part of man progresses, it will be necessary for the mind or soul to be equipped with servants in the shape of flesh and blood.

Mind, in order to develop, must be exercised; the same as one would exercise the body to acquire physical strength, consequently, the mind must have implements with which to work.

Man has not always possessed the same amount of intelligence. It is hoped that he may gain more each succeeding year.

The mind, like all else, had a beginning. In its beginning, undoubtedly a great number of life existences in the past, the mind must have occupied a body in keeping with its mental caliber. Imagine a body infinitesimally small enough to clothe the beginning of the mind or soul! Yet, however insignificant, it was adequate.

Mind in its progression is similar to a child who begins in the kindergarten, and developing sufficiently, is advanced to the first grade and so on through grammar school, high school and college; in each succeeding grade the old books are set aside and advanced ones take their place; the difference being that the child eventually graduates from college, while the mind never attains the state

25

of graduation in God's school. In each re-incarnation there is a death of the old body and a birth of the new, of a higher order, repeated numberless times during the eternal existence.

WISDOM OF THE LOWER CREATURES.

Man possesses only enough of God's wisdom to make him wonder, but is inclined to speak slightingly of the intelligence or wisdom of the so-called lower animals or creatures. There are, however, many of these so-called lower creatures, with sufficient intelligence to set an example for man, for instance:—the ant and the bee in industry; the horse for gratitude and the dog for faithfulness. That they are nearer than man to God and in constant communion with Him, that He feeds, clothes and guides them, can be proven in many ways. A cat, placed in a bag and turned loose several miles from home, will return in the time required to travel the distance. A hound, after chasing a fox twenty miles, does not retrace his circuitous route to return to his master, but elevates his nose, gives a few sniffs in the air and takes the shortest cut.

A carrier pigeon is frequently released thousands of miles from home—he immediately soars high in the air, circles about a few times and then takes a "bee-line" for his cot.

The robin hops along with his head erect; suddenly he places his bill in the earth and draws out a worm. These impulses were all the result of God-given intuition or instinct.

This Omnipotent Intelligence also directs rats to leave an abandoned ship or one about to be scuttled; warns animals to flee before a forest fire; conveys to cows, horses and other animals the knowledge of impending danger from cyclone or tornado; directs the migration of birds; the hibernation of animals and furnishes the instinct which enables these creatures to judge whether man's thoughts for them are kindly or otherwise.

Man possesses this sixth sense, intuition, in a lesser degree than creatures of the animal kingdom. The ability to make himself understood through the power of speech has retarded its development.

MENTAL DEVELOPMENT IN KEEPING WITH THE PHYSICAL.

Mental and physical development are in keeping with each other. Should you doubt this, watch the caterpillar develop into a butterfly, the tadpole into a frog. The caterpillar's mind develops to the extent that it requires another set of implements (body) with which to work, so God gives it a body in keeping with its mental caliber—one more beautiful, with which it can fly instead of crawling. The caterpillar changed the old body for the new—a necessity, a mere incident in the development of its being into one of a higher order.

The above is true of man; when he "shuffles off this mortal coil," he simply sets aside the old and is given a new vehicle that he may still do the work to which his mind is best adapted.

Man's aim in life should be to develop the best that is within him, for his state of mental development determines the stage of existence to which he progresses; at each new birth beginning his development where he left off.

The mind is never handicapped in any reasonable attainment or undertaking, and there being practically no limit to its possible development, there must be beings in some of God's numberless planets who are as superior mentally to earthly man as he is to the most insignificant earthly creature, or to beings of the infra worlds.

"A thought is an idea in transit."—*Pythagoras.*
"The laws of thought are the laws of the universe."
—*Buchner.*
"Like attracts like, therefore the thought of a thing is the prophecy of its fulfillment."
"Thought is the force that precedes and effects all the great accomplishments of mankind."
—*Bartholomew.*

THOUGHT, ORIGIN AND EFFECTS.

Mind action is thought, therefore thought emanates from the mind or soul that it may precede words and actions.

Thought produces certain minute tissue changes in the mental and physical organizations, and the continuance of normal thought tends towards perfection. Obviously, then, abnormal thought must produce the opposite mental and physical state corresponding with such thought. Since a certain line of abnormal thought has produced abnormal mental and physical conditions, it is evident that to supplant the abnormal with normal or wholesome thought will tend to produce a healthy, normal condition in both the mental and physical organizations.

Thought is energy, it is nerve force, and nerve force is as much like electricity as one can conceive.

Thought figured prominently in the Creation; doubting this, look about and point out one item of the universe which thought did not create.

31

YOUR MIND A REPRODUCTION OF YOUR MOTHER'S DURING PREGNANCY.

Leaving generalities for the time being, consider your own condition in life: Your mother's thoughts created the quality of mind which is largely responsible for the development of your body. Your mind is simply a result of the condition of hers during the pre-natal stage of your existence. God formed the warp into which your mother wove her thoughts, thereby creating the foundation of your earthly existence. Your foetal or pre-natal mind was in tune with your mother's; it was a sensitive plate for all thoughts and impressions emanating from hers during those nine months. Your plastic mind received the impress of her thoughts and will echo them as a musical string receives and reproduces sounds from strings or keys tuned to the same pitch.

It is by thought and through thought that the sins of the parents are visited upon the children of the third and fourth generations, thus making thought largely responsible for your present condition.

THOUGHT RADIATION.

Thought radiates from the mind in vibrations through the ether or atmosphere, as ripples or waves are produced in a pond or stream by throwing in a stone. The stone is a disturbing element causing vibrations or waves to pass in all directions. On the same principle is the atmosphere affected by thought, since every thought causes a certain disturbance in the brain, from which radiate the waves of thought on the ether of the atmosphere.

The velocity of thought is dependent upon the strength of the mind and the energy or nerve force expended by the person sending out such thought.

Every thought is a boomerang to the projecting mind, for all thoughts or impressions are received by minds which are in tune with the mind from which the thought emanates. The receiver returns it to the sender, thus it can not be doubted that one realizes on silent thought. Like attracts like, therefore, if one dispatches a thought of hatred, malice or treachery, the thought is transmitted to others and returned to the sender one hundred fold or more. As is the mind so is the man. As one gives so does one receive.

When one receives what is called "punishment," such punishment is not for words and actions, but for the thoughts that preceded such words and actions.

Even the little child knows that in doing a kindness it is benefited mentally, ten-fold. If one wrongs another, the abnormal thought preceding the wrong-doing will attract like thoughts. The law of retribution is always active; man realizes at once upon kindnesses extended or wrongs done.

When man arrives at the age of discretion the Great Bookkeeper opens an account with him, and the only commodity that will appear in his account is thought. Every debit item will be preceded by thought, which will have to be offset by a credit item seemingly ten times as large and this latter will have been preceded by thought. How careful one should be regarding one's thoughts, all of which find their way into the "Life Account," which only the creditor can balance. Before advancing a thought, how necessary to first consider whether or not it is kind and truthful, giving to others a "square deal," such as we, ourselves, would ask.

THE MAJORITY OF PATIENTS RESPONSIBLE FOR THEIR OWN CONDITION.

Experience proves conclusively that at least seventy-five per cent of the patients seeking treatment are responsible for their own condition, which has been produced, primarily, by abnormal thought.

The above statement will not be considered conservative by many members of the medical profession, as other statements, regarding the influence of thought upon the physical, have been doubted by them.

In justification of the statement, let us consider the cause and effect of colds. A large percentage of physical weaknesses are due to neglected colds and a large majority of colds are taken through carelessness. They are not properly guarded against. Sitting in draughts or cold rooms, failure to exchange damp clothing for dry, or wearing clothing not in keeping with the weather induces them. The foregoing colds are due to carelessness of thought which preceded carelessness of action.

The heart, lungs, stomach, intestines, kidneys, bladder, pelvic viscera and other organs may be affected by abnormal thought to such an extent as to weaken not only those parts but the entire body—the entire nervous system.

THE MIND THE CHIEF FACTOR IN THE CAUSATION OF DISEASE.

When the nervous system is weakened, thereby weakening the physical, any disease designated by a "scientific" or Latin name is liable to swoop down upon the body and take possession of it. The patient, in the majority of cases, produces the condition himself by continued abnormal thought and over-indulgences, thereby handicapping the brain.

The physician should bear in mind that muscles, ligaments, tissues, bones, etc., would be just as lifeless without the mind, as the engine without the engineer to regulate the amount of energy; that the factors of man (mind and body) are interdependent—the mind relying upon the body and the five senses (as servants) to obey its will that it may develop—the body relying upon the mind for energy and instruction, the amount of energy and quality of instruction from the mind determining largely the condition and life of the body, and that, in justice to themselves and their patients, physicians can not afford to overlook the condition of either of these factors of man when diagnosing and treating disease.

Since all parts of the body (including the five senses) are servants of the mind or soul and under its direct care and keeping, I will endeavor to demonstrate clearly by illustrations and comparisons that a large majority of the diseased conditions of these servants is caused by abnormal thinking and that the remaining conditions are due to mechanical pressure.

THE MIND THE PRIME FACTOR OF ONE'S EXISTENCE.

The medical profession should not overlook the prime factor of the patient's existence, the mind, when diagnosing a case. Mental causes could be discovered in a majority of cases, but material ones are assigned and experimental treatment given. This course may be partially due to the fact that to a patient who may be in the throes of turbulent thought, the mechanical and physical-cause arguments appeal, while the mental-cause argument will offend him. Regardless of the depleted mental condition of the patient, the physician realizes it is not wisdom to reflect upon his good (?) judgment, so he treats his patient, and whether he effects a cure or not, does he attempt to remove the mechanical or other impediment which he named as the cause for this illness? If he failed to remove or reduce that condition, was he not mistaken in his diagnosis? If the apparent mechanical disability was not the cause and he was unable to detect a mental cause, possibly he gave NATURE a chance to effect a cure.

It matters not whether the cause of disease is mental tension, mechanical pressure or otherwise, CASES SHOULD BE CORRECTLY DIAGNOSED AND THE CAUSE REMOVED BEFORE NATURE CAN RESTORE THE BODY TO A NORMAL, HEALTHY CONDITION.

Could an engineer hope to get service from pulleys, belts, bands, etc., without steam or force to operate them, if through his incompetency the energy necessary to run the machinery were impeded?

Could one's mind, as an engineer, transmit

through the nervous system to the human machinery (the body) sufficient nerve force or energy for normal service if the brain were handicapped by abnormal thought? NATURE can be handicapped in so many ways it is impossible to point out each one, but the following discourse and illustrations will serve to establish the effect of thought upon the organs and their functions.

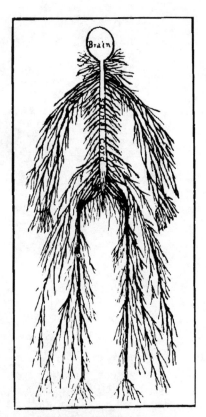

Fig. 1.
The Nervous System.
(Foundation of the Body.)

THE NERVOUS SYSTEM.

When a building is to be erected the first work considered after signing the contract is its foundation. The contractor knows the stability of the structure is dependent upon it, therefore the first part of the human structure considered will be its foundation (the nervous system), the medium through which the mind transmits thought, nerve force or energy to the body.

Fig. 1 represents the motor nervous system as it appears dissected from the human body. It is the fundamental principle, and is to the body as is the foundation of a building to the structure. Should it become weakened by a mechanical or mental impediment to the thought or nerve force which it transmits, the structure would soon warp and topple.

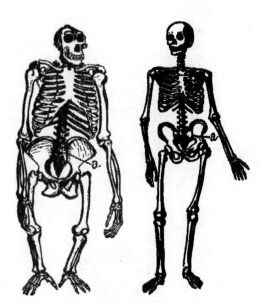

Fig. 2.
The Skeleton.
(Framework of the Body.)

THE SKELETON.

Fig. 2 represents the human skeleton and that of the gorilla; a comparison of them shows that they have the same number of bones (about 208), similar in shape and similar in arrangement. The only difference in the arrangement is that the large toe of the gorilla is at an angle to the smaller toes, while that of man is parallel.

The skeleton is the framework of the body, and is to the body as are the studding and rafters of a building to the superstructure.

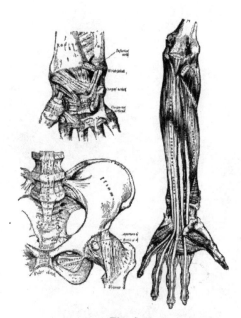

Fig. 3.
Ligament, Muscle and Tendon (Gray).
(Braces, Clap-boards and Sheathing of the Body.)

LIGAMENT, MUSCLE AND TENDON.

Fig. 3 shows the difference between ligament, muscle and tendon. Ligaments are employed in joints to hold the bones forming the joints firmly together. The upper left hand picture in Fig. 3 represents the palmar surface of the right wrist joint. In each wrist joint there are eight small bones—notice how these bones are held firmly together by ligaments which pass in every conceivable direction.

The lower left hand picture in Fig. 3 represents an anterior view of the left hip joint—a ball and socket joint. Notice how the head of the femur or thigh bone fits into the hip socket and is held there by ligaments that pass in all directions, holding, as said previously, the bones firmly in position, but allowing movement.

At the right in Fig. 3 muscles are shown, the principal muscle being the flexor profundus digitorum, flexor signifying that it flexes or bends, profundus meaning the deep muscle of the fore-

49

arm, and digitorum, the digits (the fingers), hence the name.

The fleshy part of the muscle is called the muscular part, while the tapering part is known as the tendinous portion.

The 500 muscles are attached to the frame-work of the body (the skeleton) to hold man in a normal physical condition as are sheathing and clapboards attached to the frame-work (studding and rafters) of a building for the purpose of maintaining it in a shapely condition and to prevent warping.

8

"The outer man is only an expression of his thoughts."

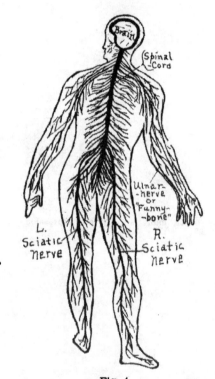

Fig. 4.
Motor Nervous System and What It Supplies.

THE MOTOR NERVOUS SYSTEM.

 Fig. 4 represents the motor nervous system and what it supplies. The motor nervous system supplies the voluntary muscles or muscles of motion, that is, those under the control of the will or mind, such as are found in the arms, hands, legs and feet. The nervous system consists of the brain and its continuation, the spinal cord. From this cord issue the forty-one pairs of principal nerves, and from these in turn the infinite number of nerves of the body, variously estimated at from ten to twenty millions. Man is a veritable bundle of ''live wires'' and the nervous system could be likened to a pipe system. The nerves are to all intents and purposes hollow, their office being to convey brain fluid to the entire body. Picture in your mind a hose-pipe system and you will then have a correct mental image of the nervous system.

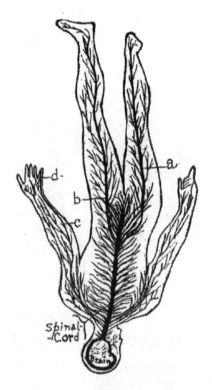

Fig. 5.
Motor Nervous System (Inverted).

MAN LIKE AN ELECTRIC LIGHTING
PLANT.

The function of the brain is similar to that of
a steam engine, dynamo or motor, and since the
object is to prove that disease in the human body
is an effect produced by either a continued mental
tension or mechanical pressure, I shall proceed
to do so by comparing man with an electric lighting plant represented by Fig. 5.

Fig. 5 is Fig. 4 inverted (turned upside down).
Let the brain represent the dynamo in which electricity is generated, and the nerves the wires which
convey the electricity to the lights, represented
by the ends of the fingers, toes, etc., in fact, all
parts of the body may be lights for our purpose,
since all parts are supplied by nerves and nerve
force.

ONLY TWO CAUSES OF DISEASE.

There are two ways of disabling this plant
(Fig. 5), either locally or generally, that is, one
light or all can be dimmed or extinguished. One
by pressing on the wire leading to that light.
Pressure upon the wire "a" will extinguish the

light to which it leads. A pressure upon "b" will have a similar effect, or a pressure upon "c" will cause a flickering of the light "d" which is supplied by that wire. The flickering of the light "d" is an effect—the cause must be found and removed before the effect; so the electrician follows the course of the wire back from the disabled or extinguished light and locates the cause at "c"— finding a pressure upon the wire or a grounded circuit. When the impediment to the wire at "c" is removed and its conductivity restored, the light "d" will burn brightly as before—we have removed the cause, thereby the effect—the cause being a pressure upon the wire between the source of supply (the dynamo) and the part supplied (the light).

All lights may be dimmed or put out by handicapping the dynamo. Under favorable conditions 100 per cent. of electricity is generated in the dynamo, but there may be an incompetent engineer in the basement, incapable of advancing the right thought in the operation of the dynamo; as a result, only 50 per cent. of the necessary electricity or energy is generated. The cause is not found to be a defect in the plant, but in the incompetency of the engineer. Supplant him by one who is competent, the dynamo will then generate a sufficient supply for the lights and their normal condition will be restored. Again the cause is removed, which was a direct handicap to the source of supply (the dynamo).

As the electric lighting plant may be disabled in two ways, locally or generally, so the human electric lighting plant (man) may be *diseased* in two ways, locally or generally, that is, mechanically or mentally.

Man is diseased locally or mechanically by pressing upon one of the nerves shown in Fig. 5. Pressure upon the sciatic nerve "a" will transmit an impulse along its entire course. A like pressure upon the sciatic nerve "b" will produce a similar diseased condition in the muscles and tissues which it supplies.

A pressure upon the ulnar nerve "c" at the elbow (better known to the laity as the "funny" or "crazy bone") will transmit an impulse to the little finger and to the inside of the ring finger which it supplies, causing lack of ease or dis-ease, proving conclusively that the parts supplied by an affected nerve will be diseased. The disease in the fingers is the effect, the pressure at the elbow the cause, and it must be removed to remove the effect. How is the cause to be removed? Shall we poultice or amputate the fingers, diet the patient or resort to drug medication? None of the above mentioned treatments would effectively remove the pressure (cause) at the elbow. Mechanical manipulation alone will remove the mechanical cause and restore the conductivity to the nerve, a normal amount of nerve force will then supply the dis-eased part with life and vitality. Another cause has been removed, which was an impediment to the nerve force between the source of supply (the brain) and the parts supplied (the fingers).

As the electric lighting plant (Fig. 5) is disabled generally (all the lights are extinguished) by handicapping the dynamo, so is the human electric lighting plant (man) *diseased* generally by handicapping the human dynamo (the brain) by abnormal thought, excesses or dissipation.

Under the heading of abnormal or uncontrolled thought should be included such mental conditions as hurry, worry, envy, anger, jealousy, hatred, "brain storms," over-mental exertion, monotony, and too long or too close application to any pursuit, while excesses or dissipation are the effect of such abnormal or uncontrolled thought. Thoughts precede words and actions, therefore all psychic or mental causes can be grouped under the heading of "abnormal thought."

Under normal conditions 100 per cent. of nerve force (thought, brain fluid, strength, energy, vitality or electricity, if you so wish to call it) is generated in the brain to supply the body. Dissipate 50 per cent. or more of the 100 per cent. in abnormal or harrowing thought, there will be a balance of 50 per cent. or less, an amount insufficient to maintain a healthy condition of the body.

By harrowing thought is meant the condition of mind wherein one continually indulges in worry, anger or any disturbing mental exertion. A great percentage of adults, of America in particular, entertain such thoughts for lengths of time sufficient to deprive them of appetite and sap their strength.

Uncontrolled thought is as dangerous as uncontrolled steam or electricity. An uncontrolled boiler or dynamo is liable to destruction; so are man's hopes and ambitions frequently wrecked by ungoverned thought, and with dreadful consequences.

A locomotive could not possibly haul a train of cars with an open valve which allowed 50 per cent. of the necessary steam to escape, nor a stationary engine hoist a load with only half the required power.

Abnormal thought affects the brain as a leakage affects the amount of water contained in a bucket. A constant dripping will soon result in depletion; stop the leakage, thereby conserving the substance.

We had first a mechanical cause with which to contend and it was removed by mechanical manipulation without effort or faith on the part of the patient, but in mental cause we have a totally different proposition with which to deal, in the removal of which the patient must be the chief factor.

The physician should point out to the patient the means by which he may rid his mind of this absorbing thought, the patient must conquer it, but co-operation is necessary.

MIND TREATED AS THE FLOWER GARDEN.

The patient's mind should be treated as the flower garden. The gardener uproots the weeds, thus saving the nutrition to be assimilated by the flowers, that they may grow and flourish. Mental weeds or excesses would drawf the mental flower and must be uprooted.

The well known axiom: "That two things can not occupy a given space at the same time," makes it evident that if uncontrolled thought is in possession of the mind, normal or natural thought can not enter.

Therefore, physicians should encourage patients to acquire a knowledge of anatomy and physiology, also of the effect of mental tension as well as mechanical pressure upon the body and its members. They should demonstrate clearly the office of the nervous system; how nerve force is generated, how dissipated; the effect of such dissipation and the importance of conserving one's nerve force and vitality.

Impress upon the patient's mind that NATURE will exact a penalty for disobedience of her laws.

Emphasize the necessity of living a life of moderation, that moderation in everything is conducive to health.

Advise patients to decline, positively, to entertain disturbing thought, it is an enemy; urge them to reason with self as with a member of their family, to exercise self-control and to treat an objectionable thought as they would an objectionable person, for the longer it is entertained the more difficult to eliminate from the mind.

PARALYSIS, APOPLEXY AND INSANITY, HOW CAUSED.

Harrowing or abnormal thought causes nervous prostration which invariably precedes paralysis, apoplexy or insanity.

Paralysis is death of the tissues produced by robbing them of nerve force.

The brain is not unlike the body; its sudden or violent exercise requires more nerve force and blood than is normal, this excess crowds its vessels, they become engorged to such an extent that one may burst, the result being called apoplexy.

Insanity is produced, generally, by concentration of thought upon one subject, not necessarily disagreeable—Religious fanatics and enthusiasts of various cults for example. Inventors frequently become unbalanced by unceasing concentration upon one subject. Thus it is evident that the mind figures prominently in maintaining health or producing disease, and is about all that really counts in man.

MAN COMPARED WITH A MODERN OFFICE BUILDING.

Abnormal thought has the same effect upon the brain and body as leakage from a tank intended to supply a building, has upon the supply.

Let Fig. 4 represent a building, and the brain a tank on the roof, filled with water to supply the building. The spinal cord would serve as the main pipe, with its branches representing the tributaries through which the water passes to the tenants. One tenant can be deprived of water by a stoppage or a break in the small pipe through which he is supplied, or all the tenants by the emptying of the tank (the brain).

This same illustration may represent the human dwelling which has but one tenant (the mind or soul). There are two grades of servants in this human dwelling; the brain being the head servant, and subservient to the mind, while the heart, lungs, stomach, intestines, kidneys, liver, arms, legs, etc., are the under-servants and dependent upon the head servant (the brain) for direction. One of the under-servants can be deprived of power to respond to this ruling force or chamberlain by a pressure or impediment to the nerve through which he should receive his directions or orders. Should the head servant or brain become disabled by excess or from other causes, a demoralization of the whole retinue of servants would result. Lack of government, confusion, disorder, and neglect would render the dwelling unfit for habitation by the master. The mind or soul would then vacate and seek another shelter.

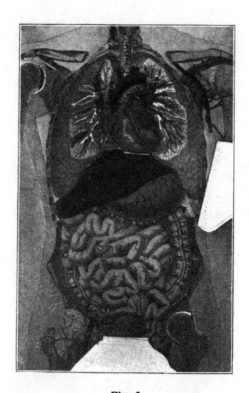

Fig. 6.
Involuntary Organs of Man.
From the "Physician's Anatomical Aid."
By permission of The Western Publishing House, Chicago.

INVOLUNTARY ORGANS OF MAN.

Fig. 6 represents some of the involuntary muscles, viz.: the heart, lungs, liver, stomach, intestines, bladder, etc., the spleen and pancreas being back of the stomach and the kidneys back of the large intestines.

These involuntary muscles which are not directly under the control of the will, are supplied by the sympathetic nervous system.

Fig. 4 represents the *motor* nervous system and the voluntary muscles which it supplies (the muscles of motion) and shows that they issue from the *sides* of the spinal cord, while the sympathetic system of nerves (Fig. 7) arises from the *anterior* portion of the spinal cord and supplies the involuntary organs in Fig. 6.

The difference between voluntary and involuntary muscles can better be explained or shown in the act of eating: Voluntary muscles are used to masticate the food, while involuntary muscles act upon the food after it is passed into the stomach or alimentary canal.

"It is the mind that maketh the body rich."
—*Shakespeare.*

"Both life and death can come in a thought."
—*Bartholomew.*

"Every physician should know or ought to know that the ailments of the body can not be cured as long as the mind is distressed. Could you get satisfactory service from a machine if there were an impediment to the force required to run the same?"
—*Bartholomew.*

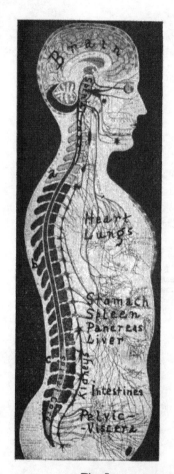

Fig. 7.
Sympathetic Nervous System.
From Eale & Taber's Anatomical Chart.
Courtesy C. W. Taber, Evanston, Ills.

SYMPATHETIC NERVOUS SYSTEM.

The nerves shown in Fig. 7, issuing from the anterior portion of the spinal cord, below the neck, are the sympathetic nerves which supply the parts represented in Fig. 6.

The sympathetic system of nerves is a subdivision of the general nervous system. The function of a sympathetic nerve, like that of a motor nerve, is to transmit impulses and nerve force.

The picture, as a whole, represents the left lateral half of the brain and spinal cord. The spinal cord, as you will notice, is a large nerve or pipe, passing down from the brain through the spinal canal; this spinal canal being formed by the twenty-four vertebrae and the sacrum. Nerve force, vitality, energy or electricity is generated in the brain and passes down through the main pipe (the spinal cord) and out through its sympathetic branches to supply the heart, lungs, stomach, intestines, liver, pancreas, spleen, kidneys and bladder, as well as through other branches to supply the eye, ear, throat, arms, legs, etc.

The parts supplied by this sympathetic system of nerves may be diseased in the same manner, locally or generally, as are the portions supplied by the motor nervous system, that is, mechanically or mentally, but direct pressure can not be produced on any of these nerves that issue from the anterior part of the spinal cord to form the sympathetic nerve system. The twelve pairs of cranial nerves arise from the upper part of the spinal cord and inside the cranium and are therefore protected by the cranium or skull.

The thoracic or chest nerves are within the chest walls of the thorax, they, together with the heart and lungs are protected by the ribs, while those inside the abdominal cavity are protected by the abdominal muscles and viscera.

SPINAL DISEASES, LAME BACKS, CAUSE OF AND EFFECTS.

Impulses may be transmitted over any of these nerves by a pressure upon the spinal cord at the point from whence they issue: Thus, pressure upon the spinal cord at "a" would transmit an impulse to the heart and lungs; a similar pressure upon the cord at "b" would affect the solar plexus, diseasing the stomach, liver, spleen and pancreas which are supplied by that plexus or net work; while pressure at "c" would transmit an impulse to the kidneys, intestines and pelvic viscera, diseasing those parts. Pressure may be produced upon the spinal cord by one or more displaced or deviated vertebrae or by a contracted condition of the spinal muscles.

A vertebra may be displaced or deviated from its normal position by a sudden wrench or strain; by occupation or by an unevenly contracted condition of the muscles and tissues surrounding the spinal cord. This contraction may be the effect of overexertion, cold or "grip" and atmospheric changes as well as by a displaced vertebra.

All muscles and ligaments are attached to bones, therefore, displace a bone and the muscles attached are placed upon a tension, and press upon the thousand and one little nerves that pass around, through and between these contracted muscles and ligaments, diseasing the part or parts supplied by the compressed nerves.

As the spinal cord fills the spinal canal, the deviation of a vertebra, muscle or tissue surrounding it, one one-hundredth part of an inch from the normal, produces a pressure upon it, and cuts off part if not all the nerve supply through it, just as pressure upon a hose-pipe diminishes or shuts off entirely the garden supply of water through the pipe.

Pressure upon the spinal cord at the point from whence issue the nerves supplying the heart, produces a diseased condition of the heart that simulates tachycardia, bradycardia and functional or organic heart trouble; if the pressure is where the impulse is transmitted to the lungs a diseased condition is produced that simulates incipient consumption, or, if there is pressure upon the main pipe from which those arise that form the solar plexus, the stomach, spleen, pancreas and liver will be affected, thus producing conditions simulating gastritis, gastralgia, dyspepsia or indigestion. If the affected nerve incapacitate the liver, the disease is known as jaundice or torpid liver. A pressure over the intestional center produces a condition that simulates constipation or the opposite condition. In the case of the kidneys—nephritis, uraemic poisoning, brights disease or diabetes will be the result.

Reducing the dislocation or relaxing the contracted muscles by careful manipulation will relieve the condition, consequently the effect.

There are two especially weak points in the spine—viz.: in the neck and the hip-joint.

The bones of the neck are very small and frail. Should a person weighing approximately 150 to 250 pounds fall upon the head, his entire weight would be upon the frail vertebrae or bones of the neck, slightly twisting one or more of them from the normal position, producing pressure upon the spinal cord. An impulse from this pressure could be transmitted to any of the cranial nerves; if to the optic, dimness of vision would be the effect;

if to the auditory nerve, deafness would be produced, and so on ad infinitum, possibly producing insanity or any of the numberless infirmities to which flesh is heir.

Generally, any affection of the cranial nerves due to pressure upon the spinal cord in the neck, is indicated by a tired feeling at the base of the brain, radiating to the shoulders, producing a desire to lean or rest the head upon something.

An impulse from this same pressure can be transmitted in the opposite direction over the pneumogastric and cardiac nerves, diseasing the heart, lungs and stomach, the organs to which these nerves lead.

The cause of derangement, which in either case results in a loss of a portion of the 100 per cent. of necessary energy, is to be found in the pressure in the neck, and must be removed before the diseased condition of the eye, ear, nose, throat, heart, lungs, etc. can be removed, as none of the organs can fulfill their mission on less than their full quota of 100 per cent. The cause is mechanical; again, manipulation is necessary to remove it, but the mechanical impediment, bear in mind, may be due primarily to *careless thought* which preceded careless action.

The other especially weak point in the spine is at the hip-joint (the junction of the hip bones with the sacrum and known as the lumbar region or "small of the back"), see Fig. 2 "a."

The hip bones are attached to each side of the sacrum by ligaments, and to the hip bones the limbs are attached in like manner. The entire weight of the trunk of the body rests upon this joint, formed by the hip bones and sacrum.

A large majority of lame backs and diseased spinal conditions are at this joint, the sacrum being forced forward upon the innominate bones (hip-bones) or the hip bone is forced backward, in some effort, possibly in lifting, or even in such a simple action as lacing a shoe. This is called by the laity a "crick in the back" or a "stitch in the hip," but diagnosed by the physician as lumbago, sciatica or rheumatism. The lumbar muscles when placed upon a tension, by displacing these bones, produce pressure upon the lumbar section of the spinal cord conveying impulses to the kidneys, intestines and pelvic viscera, diseasing those parts.

Sacrum and innominate (hip) displacements also produce pressure upon the great sciatic nerve, transmitting an impulse along its course and impeding the propulsion of nerve force to muscles which it supplies, thus disabling all organs and parts dependent upon this nerve. We have here another mechanical cause with which to contend; it

78

also requires a mechanical manipulation to remove.

The good work of one of man's organs is dependent upon the harmonious work of all the others; in fact, a man may be compared to a chain which is only so strong as its weakest link. When one link is defective so is the whole. One defective organ in the body cripples them all. By this is proved that a local cause produces, not only a local, but a general diseased condition.

HOW INHARMONIOUS THOUGHT DISEASES THE ENTIRE BODY.

A general diseased condition of the parts supplied by the sympathetic, as well as the motor nervous system, is also produced by continual indulgence in abnormal thought.

Under normal conditions the brain generates 100 per cent of nerve force or brain fluid to supply the entire body, but if by uncontrolled thought, excesses or dissipation, one dissipates the bulk of this 100 per cent of nerve force, you will readily understand that the body can not be maintained in a natural, healthy condition upon the balance of energy. There should be a tank (brain) full of energy at all times, but if one-half the brain fluid leaks out there will be only half the necessary supply remaining to pass down through the main pipe (the spinal cord) and its branches to supply the heart, lungs, stomach, intestines, liver, spleen, pancreas, kidneys, bladder, eyes, ears, nose, throat, arms, legs—in fact, the entire body; all parts of the body are trying to do normal work when supplied from a tank which is only half full of energy. The following conditions will be the result:

The eye is entitled to 100 per cent of nerve force, but if deprived of 50 per cent, dimness of vision will result; rob the auditory nerve of 50 per cent, impaired hearing or deafness is the effect; depriving the brain, itself, of 50 per cent of the necessary nerve force, produces insanity. A tired feeling is experienced at the base of the brain which radiates to the shoulders. The inability of the heart to pump the blood to all parts of the body on 50 per cent of the necessary force, produces a sluggish circulation; the lungs can not force out the carbonic acid gas (CO_2) and other impurities of the blood; the stomach can not digest the food that the nutritional substances of the same may be assimilated; the intestines can not eliminate the waste, allowing the toxic or poisonous substances to remain and be absorbed by the system. The liver is sluggish, interfering with the normal generation and flow of gall from the gall bladder into the intestines. The kidneys can not eliminate the poisonous substance which it is their office to collect, and the same is absorbed by the system. Not only do the above named organs lack the strength to functionate, but every part of the human body is robbed alike of nerve force and vitality. The mind can not enter into a conspiracy with the brain and rob the heart of 50 per cent of nerve force and still give to each of the other organs 100 per cent of energy, rob the mind and every part of the body is robbed. The muscles, ligaments, tendons and tissues of the body are just as lifeless and useless without nerve force as would be the pulleys, belts, bands, etc., of a manufacturing plant without steam to propel them. If you were operating a dynamo which generated the electricity sufficient to light a building, it would be impossible to give any particular lamp the required energy and deprive another light of a like amount, unless there were an impediment to the wire or a grounded circuit.

When all parts of the body are diseased as above, by continued abnormal thought, the condition is known as mind depletion, nerve depletion, nerve exhaustion or nervous prostration, which invariably precedes paralysis, apoplexy or insanity.

Paralysis is death of the tissues, produced by robbing them of nerve force and circulation. One's brain is not unlike the physical self; the more the brain is exercised, the greater the amount of nerve force and blood required to supply it. When the blood vessels of the brain become engorged to that extent that one of them bursts, you are then said

81

to have apoplexy; while insanity is often caused by concentration of thought upon one subject to the exclusion of all others. Religious fanatics and inventors frequently lose their mental balance by concentrating their thoughts upon one absorbing subject which has taken possession of their mind.

Abnormal thought can, if protracted, produce any and all diseases in the human body at one and the same time.

If abnormal thought is in possession of the mind, producing the diseases referred to above, it must be supplanted with normal, peaceful wholesome thought, to give NATURE a chance to repair the damages.

NATURE IS THE PHYSICIAN.

Physicians should bear in mind that NATURE is the physician, always has been, always will be, and that they are only her helpers or assistants, that it is their duty to FIND AND REMOVE THE CAUSE OR CAUSES which handicap her work, when she will effect the cure.

If thought can produce such infinite variety of diseases then our thoughts, which precede our words and actions, must have determined our present condition in life, and will determine it in the life to come.

Whether a patient's condition is due to mental tension or mechanical pressure, or both, the physician should always advise him regarding his thoughts. Guide the patient in the right trend of thought, for it is useless to give treatment, mechanical or otherwise, if he be suffering mentally. Advise the patient to control his thoughts, not to dwell on his troubles, to avoid lurid descriptions of murder or divorce trials, and all that tends to excite him. Tell him to forget the past, to live in the present and not attempt to "cross bridges" before coming to them. Explain to him that when Burns says: "Patient, cautious, self-control is wisdom's root," that he meant the controlling of one's thoughts is wisdom—that he who controls his thoughts is wise.

"Idleness is the rust that attaches to the most brilliant."

—Voltaire.

"It requires mind to accumulate great wealth and distribute it wisely, not physique."—*Jayne.*

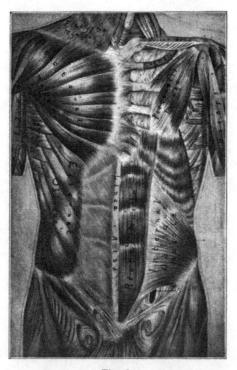

Fig. 8.
Muscles of Front of Body.
From the "Physician's Anatomical Aid."
' permission of The Western Publishing House, Chicago.

MUSCLES OF FRONT OF BODY.

Fig. 8 represents the muscles of the front of the body. On the right is shown the first layer of muscles; the pectoralis major, external oblique, etc. On the left the second layer, the rectus, pectoralis minor, internal oblique, etc. There are about 500 muscles in the human body and these muscles are attached to the surface of the bones to hold the body in position. It is through the muscles that motion is produced. The mind telegraphs nerve force (thought) to a certain set of muscles in keeping with the exertion. The muscles contract and approximate the bones to which they are attached producing motion.

A break, breach or hernia is most liable to develop at "A," owing to the thinness of the abdominal muscles at that point, and the severe strains to which they are frequently subjected.

"Character is not of the body but of the mind or soul."   *—Jayne.*

"Good thoughts are not lost though they are not practiced."

.

"Character is not of the body but of the mind or soul."   —*Jayne*.

"Good thoughts are not lost though they are not practiced."

RIBS, LIVER, STOMACH, ETC.

Fig. 9 shows the muscles as having been re-moved, exposing the exterior of the ribs, liver, stomach, small and large intestines and bladder. These, as well as the organs of the entire body, are supplied with nerves (pipes) to convey brain fluid (thought or nerve force) for the performance of their separate functions.

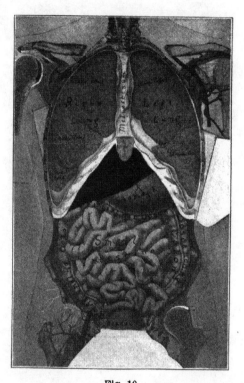

Fig. 10.
Exterior of Lungs, Etc.
From the "Physician's Anatomical Aid."
permission of The Western Publishing House, Chicago.

EXTERIOR OF LUNGS, ETC.

In Fig. 10 the ribs have been removed, exposing the exterior of the lungs, showing the left lung to consist of two lobes, while the right consists of three. Each lobe is divided and subdivided into smaller lobes called lobules. The lungs resemble elastic bags suspended in a half-inflated state in an air-tight cavity formed by the ribs (which are movable) or chest walls. The pleura or covering of the lungs is of the same formation as the inner surface of the chest or thorax that surrounds them. The pleura diminishes friction in the pleural cavity during respiration or breathing—therefore, it is a protection. The exterior of the lungs comes in contact with the inner surface of the ribs at all times, there being no space between the lungs and the inner surface of the chest.

The other organs are the same as shown in preceding Fig. 9, the function of which will be explained later.

ngs with
t colored
sages or
·eyed to

during
cted by
supply
during
tissues
blood.
·sh air
ubles
ς, and
·n by

1 the
ΆR,
bed:
·eep,
ear-

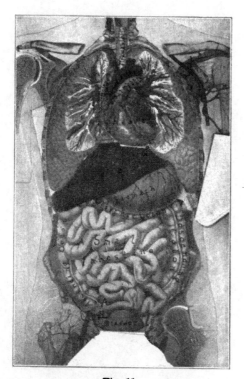

Fig. 11.
Interior of Lungs, Etc.
From the "Physician's Anatomical Aid."
permission of The Western Publishing House, Chicago.

INTERIOR OF LUNGS, ETC.

Fig. 11 represents the inside of the lungs with the heart little to left of center. The light colored lines in the lungs represent the air passages or bronchioles through which the air is conveyed to the lung tissues.

The office of the lungs is to eliminate during exhalation the impurities of the blood collected by the veins from the tissues of the body, and supply the blood with oxygen for the body tissues during inhalation. Oxygen is food or fuel for the tissues of the body and is carried to them by the blood.

The importance of breathing deeply of fresh air can not be over-estimated. Pulmonary troubles are frequently the result of shallow breathing, and of air that has been rendered devoid of oxygen by having been breathed over and over again.

Breathe like an animal—deeply, never hold the breath. Shallow breathing is induced by FEAR, in such mental conditions as you hear described: "He stood with 'bated breath." The normal, deep, fearless breather is the one who is generally fearless and courageous. "Both health and disease can come in a breath of air" the same as life or death can come in a thought, therefore, pure air for the lungs is as essential to their perfect function and the health of the body, as is pure food and kindly thought to the function of the stomach and intestines and to the life of man.

In order that the lungs may functionate normally, they must be provided with pure air from which energy can be extracted. In all parts of the United States patients suffering from pulmonary troubles are "given up," who no more need die than one within reach of food need die of starvation. Health may frequently be recovered by knowing how and what to breathe, and what and how to eat.

Many patients in the initial stages of consumption could recover their strength and vigor at home, by pursuing the same methods as practiced at a sanitarium for its treatment.

"About the most foolish thing that can be done is to try to live a Christian life without Christlike thoughts."

"No one was ever known to fool anyone other than himself."

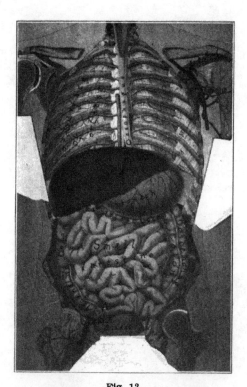

Fig. 12.
Posterior Surface of Chest, Etc.
From the "Physician's Anatomical Aid."
permission of The Western Publishing House, Chicago.

Fig. 12 shows the heart and lungs as having been removed, exposing the posterior surface of thorax or chest, also the oesophagus (gullet) through which the food is passed to the stomach.

The liver extends over the pyloric end of the stomach; it is the largest gland in the body, weighing from 50 to 60 ounces, consists of two lobes, right and left, which are subdivided into smaller lobes called lobules. The supposed function of the liver is to purify the nutritional substances of the food, conveyed to it by the portal vein (see Fig. 18). The gall or bile is generated in the liver, passed into the gall bladder, which is under the right lobe of the liver, thence into the small intestine by way of the gall duct "C," at the right of the navel or umbilicus. The gall is NATURE'S laxative—also an antiseptic and germicide. A parasite in the intestines (for example, a tapeworm) can not live where there is a free flow of gall or bile from the gall bladder or duct.

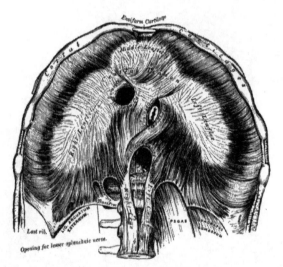

The Diaphragm (Gray).

THE DIAPHRAGM.

The diphragm (a partition or wall) is here represented, showing the under surface. The heart
and lungs are above, while the liver, stomach and
other abdominal viscera are below this partition.
It separates the chest cavity from the abdominal.
It is the chief muscle of respiration and expulsion,
is muscular at its edges and tendonous at the center. Sudden contraction of this muscle produced
by an excess of nerve force passing to it through
the phrenic nerve, causes hiccoughs. Pressure
upon the phrenic nerve decreases the amount of
energy, thus allaying the condition.

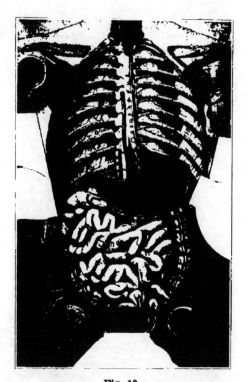

Fig. 13.
Alimentary Tract or Canal.
From the "Physician's Anatomical Aid."
By permission of The Western Publishing House, Chicago.

ALIMENTARY TRACT OR CANAL.

Fig. 13 represents the alimentary tract or canal through which food passes after mastication. The oesophagus (first part of the alimentary canal) conveys the food to the stomach through the orifice or opening known as the cardiac, and out through the second opening, the pyloric, into the small intestine, a continuation of the stomach. The first 12 inches of the small intestine is called the duodenum, the upper two-fifths of the remainder the jejunum and the lower three-fifths the ileum.

The large intestine is a continuation of the small at "A." The different parts of the large intestine are the coecum, ascending colon, transverse colon, descending colon.

The sigmoid flexure and extreme end of the lower bowel are not shown in this picture. The vermiform appendix is shown on right-hand side "B," near the junction of the small with the large intestine. Remembering that the appendix is on the right side of the abdominal cavity, will help to keep in mind the arrangement of the intestines.

WHAT, WHEN AND HOW TO EAT.

The stomach and intestines are an important link in the "human chain" and each link requires equal consideration.

After a day of physical labor the night's rest is necessary for recuperation. When the stomach has digested three square meals during the day, it should not be imposed upon by having to work all night after being gorged with the most indigestible viands. When the stomach is at work the proper rest is impossible.

The stomach and intestines are to the body what a cylinder and separator are to a threshing machine. The cylinder and separator will handle a certain amount of grain; all over its normal capacity will clog the cylinder and disable the machine. So with the human thresher, given more food than it requires, the machinery (organs of digestion, alimentation and elimination) becomes clogged or over-taxed and the surplus nutrition will be eliminated with difficulty.

The action of the intestines or bowels depends largely upon what, when and how we eat. It is not so much the quality or amount of food that furnishes energy for the human system and rebuilds wasted tissues, as it is harmony of thought. This is evidenced by the fact that different ones have fasted from 20 to 60 days; also from the fact that Japanese soldiers, carrying heavy loads, have marched and fought for several days on a daily ration consisting of a handful of rice. On a like amount of nourishment they haul a jinrikisha and its burden the entire day without loss of weight or strength. Furthermore, if the mind is in a state of inharmony, no matter how nutritious the food may be, it will not be normally digested and assimilated. How common an occurrence to be robbed of appetite at meal-time by some mental inharmony! Neither the organs of digestion, nor any other parts of the body can be expected to do normal work when those parts are suffering from robbery of nerve force or energy through the brain—due to abnormal thought or excesses.

Liquid foods are absorbed by the system, the waste being eliminated as perspiration through the skin, vapor from the lungs and urine from the kindeys. None passes through the bowels. Only the waste from solid food enters the bowels and is eliminated by them. Of a pound of beef-steak and vegetables, four-fifths will be digested and assimilated, leaving one-fifth to be eliminated by evacuation of the bowels as waste. Therefore the amount of waste or excrement eliminated by the bowels must be in proportion to the solid food of which one partakes.

NATURE ELIMINATES WASTE.

NATURE eliminates the excrement, and if helped too much, she becomes lazy and inert; if assisted *this* evening with a laxative, tomorrow she will rest complacently and say: "You helped me last evening, do the same tonight." She works faithfully if not hindered. Proper advice, manipulation and exercise will prevent the handicap.

EFFECT OF LAXATIVES.

A laxative goads the intestines to over-work, an excess of secretion (lubricant) of the inner surface of the intestines is produced, causing temporarily a diuretic condition leaving a dry inner surface of the bowel, which afterwards hinders the excrement passing through the intestines and causes directly a constipated condition. Before resorting to medicine of any sort, one should ask the question: "What is the CAUSE of my illness and will what I am about to do, or this concoction I am about to take into my stomach, remove the CAUSE? Not knowing the CAUSE, medicine is liable to go as wide of the mark as a rifleman's shot in trying to "make a bull's eye," if he were hoodwinked.

PHYSICIANS CAN NOT PRESCRIBE DIET.

Physicians can not prescribe a diet for the patient unless in serious cases, like typhoid fever, where a liquid diet is necessary. The patient knows or should know best, the food that agrees with him. The author has treated patients who have been made sick for a considerable time by a strawberry and others, apparently suffering from the same disease, who could, if they had the capacity, eat a peck and feel no ill effects, proving conclusively that "what is meat for one may be poison for another."

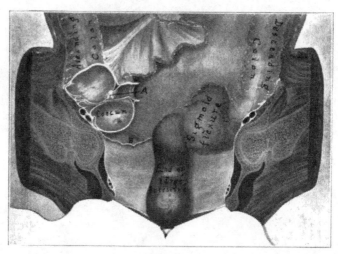

Fig. 14.
Large Intestine.
From the "Physician's Anatomical Aid."
By permission of The Western Publishing House, Chicago.

LARGE INTESTINE.

Fig. 14 represents the beginning and end of the large intestine. On the right of the abdomen "A" is where the small intestine (which has been removed) unites with the large. The ileo-coecal valve which prevents the regurgitation of the excreta, after passing into the large intestine, is at this point. The ascending colon is on the right, the descending colon, sigmoid flexure and extreme end of lower bowel on the left. The transverse colon is not shown. The appendix "B" is on the right side of the abdomen. The sigmoid flexure (S-shaped) is a sack or pouch into which the excrement of the large intestine passes, where it is subjected to a drying-out process before it is ready for elimination. Were it not for this pouch the excrement of the intestines would pass directly into the end of the large bowel and create a continual desire to defecate.

The stomach, small and large intestines are held in position in the abdominal cavity by the peritoneum and ligaments.

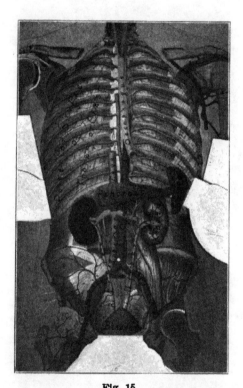

Fig. 15.
Spleen, Pancreas, Kidneys, Etc.
From the "Physician's Anatomical Aid."
y permission of The Western Publishing House, Chicago.

SPLEEN, PANCREAS, KIDNEYS, ETC.

Fig. 15 represents the spleen, pancreas, kidneys, ureters (pipes which convey the urine from the kidneys to the bladder) and bladder.

The spleen (a gland) is located on the left side of the body, back of the stomach, and is held in position in the abdominal cavity, below the diaphragm, by tissues and ligaments. Nothing is known of its function, its office is subject to conjecture, based on theory. Some physiologists claim it is a safety valve for the liver, and others, that its function is the formation of the white corpuscles of the blood.

The pancreas generates the pancreatic juice which combines with the bile or gall and flows into the intestines. This combination of pancreatic juice and bile acts upon the food in both, small and large intestines, converting the chyme of the stomach into the chyle of the intestines.

The kidneys are glands, about four inches in length and weigh from four to five ounces. The right kidney is lower than the left, on account of the liver occupying the space above it and forcing it down. The kidneys collect certain waste substances or poisonous products circulating in the blood. They also collect liquid substances direct from the alimentary tract when taken in large quantities. Excess liquids do not pass into the blood and tissues, but are taken up directly by the kidneys and passed off as urine through the ureters (pipes) to the bladder.

Water should be taken in sufficient quantity to flush the kidneys, as the bulk of liquid waste is passed through and eliminated from the system by them, especially in winter when less is passed off through the tissues by evaporation, sweat or perspiration.

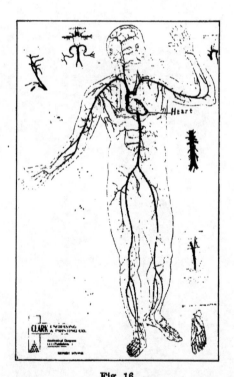

Fig. 16.
The Arterial System.
Through courtesy of The Clark Engraving & Printing Co.,
Milwaukee, Wis.

ARTERIAL SYSTEM.

Fig. 16 represents the arterial system, which in formation is similar to the motor nervous system. As Fig. 4 shows all the principal nerves arising from the spinal cord, so Fig. 16 shows that all the principal arteries arise from one main artery which extends from the top part of the heart to the branches which extend down either leg.

The heart, an organ about the size of one's doubled hand, is here shown as the head of the arterial system; it is a pump that forces the blood to all parts of the body through the arteries that the nutriment and oxygen of the blood may be deposited in the tissues. The blood, pumped to all parts of the body through the arteries, is returned to the heart through the veins.

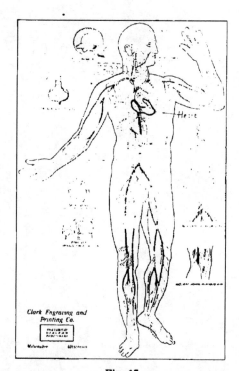

Fig. 17.
The Venous System.
Through courtesy of The Clark Engraving & Printing Co.,
Milwaukee, Wis.

VENOUS SYSTEM.

The superior vena cava and its branches (Fig. 17) collect the blood above, while the inferior vena cava (large vein) and its branches collect that below the heart and return it to that organ. Thus the heart pumps or rams the pure blood through the arteries, carrying nutrition and oxygen to the tissues, while the veins, after the nutritional substances of the arterial blood is deposited in the tissues, return to the heart the waste, toxic and poisonous substances collected; in other words, return the impure blood to be purified, revivified and sent on its journey as before.

"The best of things beyond their measure cloy."
                                    —*Pope.*
"A man's prosperity depends largely upon his health."   —*Common Sense.*
"Checking useless expenditures will enable you to draw a check for necessary ones."
"Not the possession of mcney, but to *Know Thyself* spells wealth."   —*Bartholomew.*

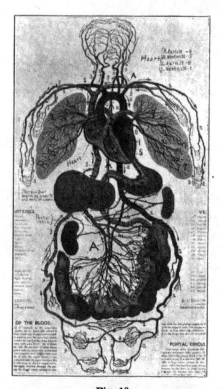

Fig. 18.
Organs of Digestion and Circulation.
From the "Physician's Anatomical Aid."
permission of The Western Publishing House, Chicago.

ORGANS OF DIGESTION AND CIRCU-
LATION.

Fig. 18 is a distorted picture, that is, the organs of digestion and circulation are not represented in their normal positions. The picture represents a combination of the arterial and venous blood systems, and is arranged principally to make the first two preceding pictures clearer and to show how the blood circulates, carrying the nutritional substance of the food through the body, and how the blood is pumped by the heart to all parts of the body and is by this same action forced to return to the heart through the veins.

WHY FOOD IS NECESSARY.

The organs of digestion have been described, also the course food takes after it passes into the alimentary canal. The question may be in order: For what purpose is food taken into the system and what becomes of it? Food is necessary, since from it, in conjunction with the air we breathe, is formed the nutriment of the blood to rebuild waste of tissues incident to oxidation. Oxidation is due to exercise of whatever nature or however slight. There is also a constant liberation of energy in the production of muscular work and in the evolution of heat, going on in the body, consequently the various tissues of the body, like a machine, are subject to wear and tear. The waste product, due to disintegration of the tissues and to combustion, are eliminated, by the lungs as carbonic acid gas (CO_2)—through the skin as perspiration and through the kidneys and bowels as urine and excrement, as has been previously stated. To make good the above loss, food is required.

Blood consists of white and red corpuscles and other solid bodies or tissues floating in a liquid medium; the quality of the blood depends principally upon the nature of the food taken into the alimentary tract, and the purity of the air into the lungs.

HOW FOOD IS DIGESTED AND ASSIMILATED.

By referring to Fig. 18 and reading carefully the following paragraphs you will understand how the nutritional substances of food are separated and conveyed to the blood vessels to combine with the blood.

Food should be thoroughly masticated and mixed with the saliva, which is an alkaline substance. It is then passed into the stomach where it is acted upon by the gastric juice (an acid)

changing the food into a substance called chyme,
thence into the small intestine where it is acted
upon by the bile and pancreatic juice which
change the substance (chyme) into chyle. The
amount of nutriment extracted depends largely
upon the fundamental work of properly chewing
the food and one's mental condition.

The arrows in the alimentary tract (Fig. 18)
show the course of the food in passing through the
stomach, small and large intestines.

The double-headed arrows show course and direction taken by the nutrient substances of the food
after it seeps through the walls of the stomach,
small and large intestines to be transported by the
portal vein and thoracic duct to the inferior and
superior venae cavae (large veins) to become part
of the blood.

The nutrient substances of food seep through
the walls of the stomach and intestines and are
taken up by the tributaries of the portal vein
(shown in Fig. 18) namely: The splenic (from
the spleen), the gastric (from the stomach) and
the superior and inferior mesenteric (from the
walls of the small and large intestines). These
four veins or tributaries of the portal vein collect
the bulk of the nutrient substances from the food
as they seep through the stomach and intestinal
walls, and convey them to the portal vein, which
in turn conveys them to the liver. In this organ

the nutrient substances of the food are subjected to a purifying process and then passed through the hepatic vein of the liver into the inferior large vein (the inferior vena cava) thus reaching the blood and becoming part of it.

The nutrient material intended for the system and not collected by the portal system, is collected by the lacteals and passed into the thoracic duct (lower "A") which conveys the same to the left sub-clavian vein (upper "A"), thence into the superior vena cava where it becomes part of the blood and passes to the heart.

HOW THE BLOOD CIRCULATES.

The following is a description of the course which the blood takes from the time it leaves the heart until it returns to it.

The arrows in the heart, arteries and veins show the course taken by the blood after leaving the left ventricle (1) until it is returned to the heart.

There are four cavities or chambers of the heart, the right. (4) and the left auricles (8) and the right (5) and left ventricles(1). When the heart contracts or beats, the blood is forced out from the left ventricle (1), passing through the arteries (2) to all parts of the body. The four cavities of the heart contract almost simultaneously, the left ventricle (1) emptying when it contracts, filling when it relaxes or dilates. From the left ventricle (1) the blood is pumped or forced out through the arteries (represented by the dark lines in Fig. 18) which carry the pure blood to all parts of the system through which they and their infinite number of branches course.

The arterial blood deposits the oxygen and nutrient substances it contains in the tissues of the body (which may be either bone, muscle, ligament or tendon) to combine with them. As the blood seeps or oozes through the tissues it collects the waste products or impurities, passing the same into the veins (3) which convey the impure blood back to the right auricle of the heart (4). The inferior vena cava and its branches collect the impure blood below the heart, while the superior vena cava and its branches collect the impure blood above the heart and convey the same to the heart. Both these large veins empty into the right auricle (4) of the heart, while the blood when leaving the heart is forced out from the left ventricle (1). Veins are called the sewers of the body, because they carry away the waste products from the different tissues of the body.

The blood returned to the right auricle (4) by the large veins is passed to the right ventricle (5), thence through pulmonary artery (6) to the lungs (7) where it remains until exhalation eliminates the carbonic acid gas (CO_2) and inhalation supplies the oxygen for absorption by the blood, when it is said to be purified or reoxygenated, and then passed from the lungs (7) to the left auricle (8), thence to the left ventricle (1) from whence it is again pumped out into the system.

One-thirteenth of the body's weight is blood, which makes the circuit through the arteries and back to the heart through the veins every forty seconds, consequently a healthy condition depends absolutely upon an equal or normal circulation, while abnormal circulation is invariably accompanied by a diseased condition. If the circulation is normal, one may, with safety, visit any hospital where contagious diseases are treated, without fear. Why? Because when the blood circulates normally or equally, it immediately surrounds, destroys and removes (much as rats would surround and devour a piece of cheese) the so-called contagious germs, impurities or waste, communicated to the visitor by way of the lungs or stomach or absorption through the skin.

CANCERS, TUMORS AND GROWTHS, HOW FORMED.

Circulation as well as the caliber of the blood vessels is governed by the vaso motor nerves (vessel-moving nerves) that pass to the walls of the blood vessels, hence it follows that a defective general circulation is caused by handicapping the dynamo or brain which is at the head of the nervous system, thus producing a nervous collapse and placing the system in a condition susceptible to disease. Cancers, tumors and growths are liable to form when the physical condition is as described above.

These diseases are a result of depleted physical condition and sluggish circulation; the lungs, bowels, kidneys and excretory glands are inactive, thus allowing the poisonous substance, which it is their office to collect and eliminate, to remain in the system.

In poor circulation the blood fails to flow freely through the firmer tissues of the body on account of the weakened condition of the heart. Some minute particles (of which the blood consists) find lodgment at some point, say upon the breast, and other particles are deposited at the same point on account of the obstruction, forming into a growth and is, by the "specialist," diagnosed as a tumor or cancer.

On the same principle drift-wood is deposited in a shallow or sluggish stream where the current is not sufficiently strong to carry it away. One piece of drift-wood finds lodgment upon the bank, another is deposited by its side, thus an obstruction is formed. Dearth of water placed it there, and water alone will remove it when the current becomes normal.

It is the office of the blood to remove the bodily obstruction in like manner, and when the circula-

139

tion is perfected in and about the growth, as well as through the body, this will have been accomplished. But the fact should be borne in mind that if the patient is suffering mentally it is utterly useless to treat him mechanically or medicinally until such mental lesion is removed. The mental lesion or cause not only hinders physical progress, but is an impediment in all the pursuits of life.

BLOOD TO THE BODY WHAT WATER IS TO A BUILDING.

Blood is to the body what water is to a building or city. The combined arterial and venous systems (Fig. 18) are similar to the water and sewer pipe systems of a large, modern building. If a water pipe is broken or occluded, the part of the building to which the pipe leads will be deprived of water. If the pump is broken which forces the water to all parts of the building, then the entire building will be rendered unfit for occupancy, as the sewage can not be carried off without its aid. The same untenantable condition will be produced if the sewer system is defective and the waste and poisonous products of the building accumulate.

The human building (man) can be rendered unsanitary in like manner. If the arterial circulation is impeded by a direct pressure upon the vessels, or by robbing the heart (the force-pump) of energy by indulgence in abnormal thought or by an impediment to the nerve force supplying same, then the tissues of the body will be deprived of the life-giving nutrition which would have been deposited in them by the blood.

Or, if there be an obstruction to the venous circulation, hindering the elimination of the waste products formed in the system and which it is the office of the veins to collect and eliminate, then disease will take possession of and invade the system.

The obstruction, as in all the foregoing instances, is oftener the result of abnormal thought than of physical origin. Advise the patient to avoid thinking of his troubles; suggest to him forgetfulness of an unpleasant past and that it is sufficient to live in the present, without having to overcome imaginary obstacles. Don't "cross bridges" before coming to them. Impress upon the patient's mind that his strength is only sufficient to enable him to bear the burdens of the day, not of the ages to come. Apropos of this Jefferson says: "How much pain the evils have cost us that have never happened."

MODERATION IN ALL THINGS NECESSARY.

The foregoing, explaining the effect of thought upon the circulation and general health, should impress the reader with the importance of protecting the storehouse of energy and giving it the same

141

consideration as the bank account, also with the fact that over-indulgencies are the outcome of abnormal thinking, and make him realize the importance of adopting for a motto "moderation in all things." It is necessary that every one become better acquainted with Self—know how his nerve force is generated, how dissipated, the effects of such dissipation and the importance of conserving or saving one's nerve force or vitality, thus protecting the Vital Bank Account, for without a good Vital Bank Account he can not make and maintain a full Cash Account.

There is probably no living person who has not, at some time, been possessed by a harrowing thought that robbed him of his energy and vitality, and when freed from it, wondered what had been worrying him. Has he ever realized on one per cent of his disagreeable anticipations? Probably not, but a check has been cashed by the Bank of Vitality, upon which no value in dollars and cents can be placed, and can only be estimated in loss of nerve force and the inharmonious conditions which result.

He drew, knowingly, a check in favor of some one for a wrong done himself.

He should bear in mind that the greatest amount of capital that he can have in his Vital Bank is 100 per cent, and that he can not have the surplus in this vital bank that there is in some cash bank accounts.

He should remember that when the bank of vitality is partly depleted, it should be repleted by economy of nerve force, as the cash bank account is replenished by saving the cents and dollars, that health is wealth, also that a brim-full storehouse, the result of pure, wholesome and fearless thoughts, is priceless.

"Moderation in all things should be the motto of mankind."   —*Bartholomew*.

"He who reigns within and rules his passions, desires and fears is more than a king."—*Marshall*.

"That which is unworthy of perpetuity should not be transmitted to children."

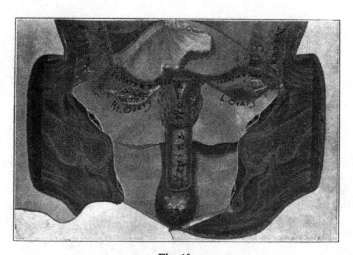

Fig. 19.
Female Pelvic Viscera.
From the "Physician's Anatomical Aid."
By permission of The Western Publishing House, Chicago.

FEMALE PELVIC VISCERA.

Fig. 19 represents the extreme end of the lower bowel or large intestine, interior of vagina, fallopian tubes, womb and ovaries. In the right ovary are shown the graffian follicles, one of which ripens every 28 days and bursts, passing the ovum off through the fallopian tubes to be eliminated through the uterus and vagina. During this time (menstruation) the uterus or womb becomes internally congested and several ounces of blood or toxic substance is eliminated. The graffian follicles of the ovary continue to ripen until the menopause (change of life) when they are exhausted. The change of life occurs later with women who have borne children. This is accounted for by the fact that the mother does not menstruate from the time of conception until from three to twelve months after confinement or labor. It is perfectly natural that women should bear children and God has made this provision, that while supplying sustenance to the offspring, she lose none necessary to her own well being.

147

"Thought is ·a force a thousand times more pow-
erful than bullets and boyonets."

"The mothers of great men and women deserve
equally as much, if not more honor, than the great
men and women themselves."

—*Bartholomew.*

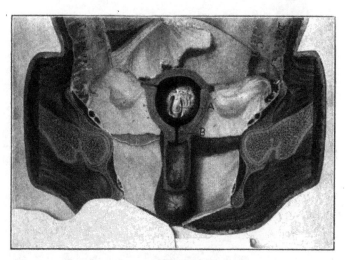

Fig. 20.
Beginning of Gestation (Conception).
From the "Physician's Anatomical Aid."
By permission of The Western Publishing House, Chicago.

BEGINNING OF GESTATION.

Fig. 20 represents the condition of the womb soon after conception. A sac, called the placenta, forms around the germ, embryo or foetus "A," and immediately the uterus or womb begins to enlarge, accommodating itself to the condition, forcing the mouth of the womb "B" lower into the vagina.

In the above and the two succeeding pictures the small intestines are not shown.

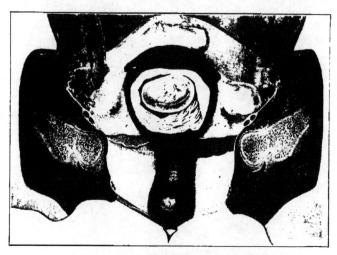

Fig. 21.
Three Months After Conception.
From the "Physician's Anatomical Aid."
By permission of The Western Publishing House, Chicago.

"One's characteristics are in keeping with one's mother's mind during pre-natal life."—*Bartholomew*.

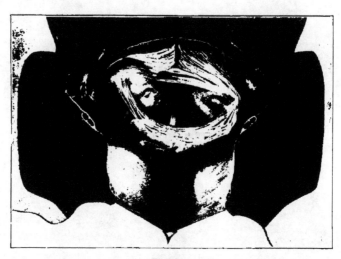

Fig. 22.
Seven Months After Conception.
From the "Physician's Anatomical Aid."
By permission of The Western Publishing House, Chicago.

SEVEN MONTHS AFTER CONCEPTION.

Fig. 22 shows stage of development of the foetus seven months after conception. The umbilical vein and artery are shown in connection with the placenta which surrounds the foetus. The placenta supplies the foetus with blood which is received from the mother's system thus taking the place of the heart and lungs, since in the entire pre-natal state these organs are inactive; when the air comes in contact with the foetus during labor or confinement, they begin their work. The air has a stimulating effect upon the child and produces respiration or action of the heart and lungs. This fact alone makes it necessary that there should be a head presentation in labor in order to avoid suffocation.

"Noble thoughts make the foundation for noble manhood." —*Segno.*

"Be the kind of a parent you would have your children become."

"Homes are built, not of stones, but of pure and wholesome thoughts." —*Bartholomew.*

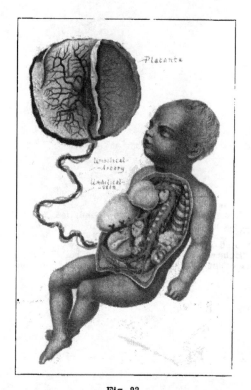

Fig. 23.
Child and Placenta.
From the "Physician's Anatomical Aid."
y permission of The Western Publishing House, Chicago.

CHILD AND PLACENTA.

Fig. 23 represents the child after delivery or birth and before the umbilical vessels have been severed. In it is observable the placenta, which surrounded the child when in the womb, and performed the offices of heart and lungs before birth or during gestation.

PRE-NATAL INFLUENCES.

When explaining the workings of the organs of the body, it is not out of place to again suggest that the trend of the mother's thoughts during its pre-natal life is directly responsible for her child's mental, moral and physical condition, and that the post-natal education would be less strenuous if the pre-natal conditions and surroundings were considered scientifically.

There is no doubting the fact that the embryological or pre-natal stage is of the utmost importance. During this period the foundation is built, and the different circumstances attending the development of each foetus account for the difference in dispositions, minds and habits of

161

children of the same family. The environments and conditions by which the mother is surrounded during pregnancy with one child usually differ materially from those of all others.

The mother can do much to shape and control the mental and physical condition of her offspring. To her state of mind during the stage of gestation is often traceable the traits of the child, whether they be those of the criminal, genius or saint.

Many an artist's mother has been known to have been a great admirer of nature and art.

Napoleon's mother was on the battle field with her husband the greater part of her son's prenatal life.

Every mother whose offspring shows special mental or physical development, whether for good or evil, can recognize the influence or cause that produced the effect.

The environment of the mother during gestation should be such as to afford her peace of mind —harmony of thought.

None but pure and wholesome thoughts should be exchanged between the parents or entertained at time of conception and during gestation, that the child may inherit a mind that will reflect credit upon them.

The certainty of the father's thought affecting the mind of the foetus, through the mind of the mother, is evidenced from the fact that when congenial parents have lived together for years, their minds and thoughts are similar, that is, their minds are in tune with each other. Each mind is a receiver or sensitive plate, to a certain extent, for the other's thoughts so that when thoughts emanate from the mind of one, whether good or bad, these thoughts are transmitted to the mind of the other parent intuitively, never failing to influence the mind of the foetus. These thought vibrations are received as impressions—as intuitions.

If, at the time of and after conception, the father entertains treacherous or deceptive thoughts, they cannot be hidden from the mother. If deceptive thoughts emanate from the mind of the mother, the father receives them intuitively.

"As a person thinketh, so is he." As is the mother's mind during the period of gestation, so will be the mind of the child.

The foregoing is true, not only of human mothers, but of all mothers throughout the animal kingdom.

When I was quite young my parents purchased a Morgan mare, after eating her hay and grain, she would devote her time to kicking the side of the stall or stable door. Her daughter, granddaughter and great grand child were just as anxious (when not provided with hay and grain) to kick down the same stable door as was their ancestor, showing how, through thought, the habits and ways of ancestors are "handed down" or inherited by the children of the third and fourth generations.

On account of lack of mental development and speech to clothe their thoughts, animal thought is not as varied as that of man. They think and act in grooves, transmitting this same line of thought to their progeny, which accounts for the continuation of the same characteristics, both of appearance and actions in animals of any given specie. This is exemplified by cats catching mice, setters and pointers locating game, hounds chasing rabbits and foxes, birds going south in winter and returning in summer—all following the same line of thought as their ancestors.

A child conceived in sin and gestated in crime seldom escapes the natural consequence—a life of crime. This statement can be proven by an examination of the records of criminologists, wherein it is shown that criminal mothers have been the progenitors of a large majority of degenerates, and the antecedents of from 400 to 500 beings who have led criminal lives are given, showing their criminal inheritance.

There is an old saying that "blood will tell," but it is not the blood that tells—it is the mind that tells.

Could parents read a record of their children from 10 to 40 years after birth and in that record note a list of crimes committed by them, only a very small percentage would take unto themselves the blame for those crimes, and the rest would doubtless say: "their children got into bad company and were led astray." Why did they get into bad company? Criminal instincts were implanted or woven into their minds prior to birth and they sought companionship of their kind.

So it naturally follows that crime has the same attraction for these children as water for a duck, it is an inherited tendency, a natural possession.

Many criminals are serving time for offences for which their parents should have been held responsible!

In many cases the parents or their ancestors should have been executed instead of the poor fellow who received the sentence!

Parents should remember that it is more creditable to have a good descendant than a good ancestor, and that the minds of their children are reflections or reproductions of theirs during the pre-natal life.

PRUDERY A CRIME.

When the home is blest with a "little visitor" the parents' work is just begun—only the foundation has been constructed, after which the good work should be continued by giving the best advice. Parents should give their children the benefit of such of their life experiences as may be profitable to them. Make companions of them and invite their confidence.

Many a girl has been made an invalid for life through the prudishness and carelessness of her parents who thought it a crime to give her information regarding the care necessary at puberty (beginning of menstruation) and after-life.

Parents should realize that prudery is a crime —that it is wrong to withold knowledge from their children that will help them to protect their mental, moral and physical being.

"In our mind's eye we see success on the hilltop; we can reach it with steadfast purpose and clean thoughts to help us in the climb."—*Bartholomew*.

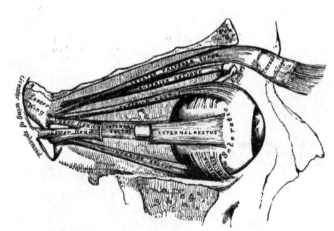

Fig. 24.
Muscles of Right Eye.   (Gray)

MUSCLES OF RIGHT EYE.

Fig. 24 represents the right eye and muscles of same (six in number). Every tissue of the eye, as well as the eye-ball, is supplied with nerves and nerve force, as are all other tissues of the body. Four and one-half pairs of cranial nerves supply the eyes, which are one-ninth the nervous system.

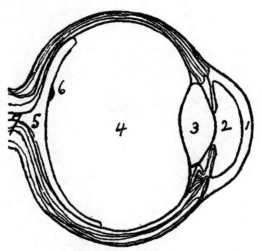
Fig. 25.
Tissues of Eye.

TISSUES OF EYE.

Fig. 25 represents the different tissues of the eye.

"1" represents the cornea which is in front of the eye, similar to the crystal of a watch. The cornea is a clear, transparent, hard tissue substance and forms one-sixth the covering of the eye-ball. The sclerotic coat forms the other five-sixths of the covering.

"2" represents the aqueous humor. It is a clear, watery fluid which fills the space between the cornea and crystalline lens. The iris divides it into two compartments.

"3" represents the crystalline lens. It is a firm, transparent muscle, capable of increasing or decreasing its convexity by the muscles of accommodation, which are shown in the upper and lower extremities of the lens.

"4" represents the vitreous humor, which is a transparent, gelatinous mass, closely resembling the white of an egg. It occupies the space back of the lens, that is, the large cavity in the rear of the eye.

The cornea, aqueous humor, crystalline lens, and vitreous humor are the refracting media of the eye, that is, they refract or break the rays of light so that they are focused on the retina and transmitted to the brain.

"5" represents the retina, a very sensitive or nervous membrane upon which the rays of light or images are focused and transmitted to the brain by the optic nerve. The point of greatest sensitiveness on the retina is known as the "yellow spot" (6).

"7" represents the optic nerve of which the retina is an expansion. This nerve connects the eye with the brain. The images which are reflected upon the retina are transmitted to the brain by this nerve (the optic).

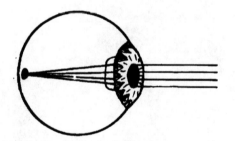

Fig. 26.
Normal or Perfect Eye (Emmetropia).

NORMAL OR PERFECT EYE.

Fig. 26 represents a normal or emmetropic eye, one in which all rays of light are focused upon the the retina. Only one per cent. of the adults of the United States have perfect or emmetropic eyes. The tissues of the eye can be likened to a stereopticon (magic lantern); the cornea and crystalline lens to the focusing lens; the retina to the screen upon which objects are reflected to be transmitted over the optic nerve to the brain and perceived by the mind.

"The measure of your thought is the measure of your success."

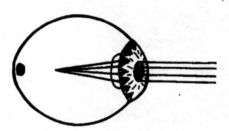

Fig. 27.
Nearsighted Eye (Myopia).

NEAR-SIGHTED EYE.

Fig. 27 represents a near-sighted eye or what is generally termed "myopia." In this condition the rays of light are focused at an imaginary point in front of the retina, due to over-convexity of the cornea. The eye-ball is bulged backward, forcing the eye forward and outward, giving the eye a prominent appearance, which you have doubtless noticed in near-sighted people. The name "near-sighted" results from the necessity of bringing the object nearer to the eye to focus the rays of light upon the retina. A concave lens is used to correct this defect as it scatters the rays of light sufficiently to allow of their being focused on the retina. In this condition there is a tendency to nearly close the eye when looking at an object.

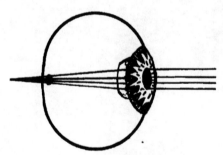

Fig. 28.
Farsighted Eye (Hypermetropia).

FAR-SIGHTED EYE.

Fig. 28 represents a far-sighted eye (scientifically called Hypermetropia). You will notice this is a condition in which the eye-ball or cornea is flattened. The rays of light are focused at an imaginary point back of the retina. The cornea and crystalline lens are not strong (convex) enough to break the rays of light so that they will be reflected or focused on the retina.

Glasses with convex lenses are necessary, in this condition, to sufficiently collect the rays of light that they may be focused on the retina and transmitted to the brain.

The far-sighted person generally has vertical wrinkles between the eyes, from squinting in an effort to see near-by objects.

In old sight, which begins about the age of forty in the normal eye, the cornea becomes flattened or rather less convex. At this time the muscles of accommodation lose their expansile and contractile power. The patient then begins to hold his reading matter farther away from the eye, that a clearer vision may be had. A tension upon the tissues and muscles of the eye when the patient is reading dissipates nerve force and he soon becomes depleted physically, owing to the constant strain. Glasses should be worn for reading, if not for other purposes, by the majority of mankind at the age of forty or over.

The nervous system may be depleted by a leakage of nerve force through the eyes, just the same as a steam engine can be deprived of power by a leakage from an open valve. Proper attention to the defect in the eye, fitting glasses that will correct it will prevent the drain on the nervous system and eliminate a menace to both the mental and physical organizations.

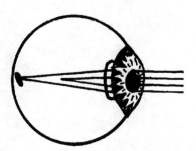
Fig. 29.
Astigmatic Eye (Astigmatism).

ASTIGMATIC EYE.

Fig. 29 represents an astigmatic eye (astigmatism) which means "without a point," that is, the rays of light as they pass through the different meridians of the eye are not focused at the same point, showing that there is more convexity in one meridian of the cornea than in the one to which it is at right angles. We will say, for instance, that the two outside rays of light enter in the vertical or 90th meridian—you will notice that they are focused on the retina, while the two middle rays enter the eye at the 180th meridian (which is at right angles to the 90th meridian) are focused at an imaginary point in front of the retina, therefore a distorted image is reflected upon the retina and transmitted to the brain.

The derivation of the word "astigmatism," is stigma, meaning a point. Astigma, meaning without a point. This condition is due to an inequality of curvature of the different meridians of the cornea.

189

My experience in treating and testing eyes convinces me that a majority of the cases of astigmatism is congenital (from birth), but may readily be the result of injury or disease, and may accompany either a near-sighted or a far-sighted condition.

In order to give normal vision to an astigmatic eye, a spherical lens must be combined with a cylindrical.

"Lose this day loitering, 'twill be the same old story
Tomorrow, and the next more dilatory,
Each indecision brings its own delays,
And days are lost lamenting o'er lost days.
Are you in earnest? Then seize this very minute,
What you can do, or think you can, begin it;
Once begun, and then the mind grows heated,
Begin it, and the work will be completed."—*Goethe*.

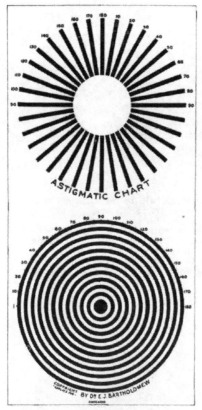

Fig. 30.
The Author's Astigmatic Chart.

THE AUTHOR'S ASTIGMATIC CHART.

Fig. 30 represents a chart of especial value to oculists and physicians in determining the axial meridian in astigmatism. It is absolutely correct. The patient PROVES the correctness of the test. Saves time. Saves nerve force of the patient. No computations necessary to determine the meridian at which axis of cylinder should be placed in trial frame, thus avoiding mistakes, so frequent, by oculists when testing for axial meridian. The accuracy and value of this chart is due to the unique arrangement of numbers on the Wheel and Disc and to the combination of the Wheel and Disc in one chart.

The merits of this chart can not be determined by this miniature picture. Every physician should possess one of the charts that he may (at a glance) test his own, as well as his patient's eyes for astigmatism, since a large majority of mankind is afflicted with it. The simplicity of the chart enables a physician to determine instantly whether or not a patient's glasses are adapted to the condition of his eyes.

TREATMENT OF THE EYES.

The abnormal conditions of the eye known as near-sighted, far-sighted and astigmatic, are malformations of the eye-ball or tissues thereof and will not yield to manipulation or medicinal treatment. These conditions can be corrected only with lenses adapted to the condition of the eye.

Four and one-half pairs of cranial nerves supply the eyes and tissues around them—four and one-half pairs of the forty-one pairs that issue from the spinal cord, or one-ninth the nervous system.

It is thus evident that the nervous system can be depleted very quickly by a leakage of energy due to imperfect vision. A large percentage of the pains about the head arise from this source.

Many headaches are caused by reading without glasses when they are needed, or by reading with glasses which are not adapted to the condition of the eyes (that is, "mis-fits"). From this source a permanent weakened condition of the organ may result.

People with defective eyes who have never worn glasses adapted to their condition, can not imagine the comfort and relief afforded by glasses fitted to relieve them of this nerve strain.

A correct test and examination of the eyes is just as essential to determine what is necessary to be done to perfect the vision, as a correct diagnosis is to the removal of the cause of disease.

Since a depleted condition of the nervous system can be caused by defective vision, the medical profession will understand the importance of possessing a thorough knowledge of the eye—how to examine it for diseased conditions, as well as to test and prescribe lenses adapted to its condition.

One of the most important of our senses is sight. It is by sight that we judge of place, size, distance, and locate objects around us. It enables us to accomplish with certainty and ease things which would be impossible, were it not for the information afforded by one of the choicest gifts of God. Time and money spent in caring for the valuable organ of sight is well spent.

Physicians should look as carefully to the condition of their own eyes as to those of their patients.

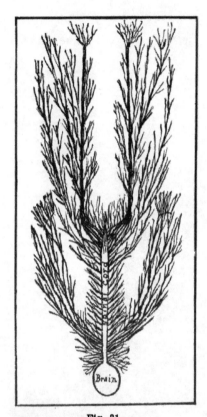

Fig. 31.
Man's "Nerve Skeleton." (Inverted).

MAN LIKENED TO A TREE, PLANT OR SHRUB.

I am keeping the nervous system before you lest you forget that it is the foundation of the body, that it is the medium through which the Almighty provides the body with nerve force, energy, vitality, strength.

To show the striking resemblance of this nervous system, when inverted, to that of a plant, tree, or shrub, since the life of a plant and that of man are similar, I will let the brain represent the roots of the plant or tree; the spinal cord and its branches, the pores which convey the sap up through the trunk to the branches.

The growth of this plant may be interfered with in two ways: locally and generally; locally, by bending or breaking one of the branches, thus destroying the conductivity of the pores supplying that particular branch; generally, by lifting the roots out of the ground or earth, thus depriving it of energy and nutrition, consequently of life.

In like manner the human plant (man) may be diseased; locally or generally, that is, mechanically or mentally; locally, by interfering with the conductivity of a nerve leading to any of its parts; generally, by handicapping the source of nerve supply (the brain) by abnormal, uncontrolled or absorbing thoughts.

Since man is a superior order of plant life and governed by the same Eternal, All-prevading Force, then fresh air, sunshine and contact with the earth are just as essential to him as to the plant, tree or shrub that grows in the field.

MAN LIKENED TO A TELEGRAPH SYSTEM.

Man may also be likened to a complicated telegraphic system, in which comparison we will use Fig. 31.

The brain represents the main office from which all orders or messages are dispatched.

Thoughts are the messages which are passed out or transmitted over this main line (the spinal cord) and its branches to the different parts of the body to which these wires lead.

The mind or soul is the telegrapher who uses the brain as a key-board to transmit thought messages over the wires to the different parts of the human telegraphic system.

This telegraphic system can be crippled in two ways: locally or generally; locally, by a break or impediment to any of these wires, destroying its conductivity, thus rendering useless that part of the telegraphic system beyond the break or obstruction, or by a careless or incompetent operator sending out incorrect messages—the frequent cause of collisions and disasters. The general or entire system can be paralyzed by the current being cut off or lack of operators at the main switchboard.

As this telegraphic system is crippled or disabled in two ways, so is the human telegraphic system (man) diseased in two ways: by an obstruction or an impediment to any of these nerves or by defective mental messages.

These mental messages (thought) precede words and actions, therefore the present condition in life is the result of thought. The future condition in this life and the life to come depends upon thought, that is, the messages of thought which are dispatched from this main office (the brain) by the mind or soul, which is the telegrapher.

It is upon these messages of thought that health, happiness and success largely depend.

"A single fact is worth a carload of argument."
"It nettles one that truth should be so simple."
—*Goethe.*
"First, keep thyself in peace and then shalt thou be able to pacify others." —*Kempis.*
"He that studyeth revenge keepeth his own wounds green, which otherwise would heal and do well."
"A man who does not know how to learn from his own mistakes, turns the best schoolmaster out of his life." —*Beecher.*
"If we have not quiet in our own minds, outward comforts will do no more for us than a Golden Slipper for a gouty foot." —*Bunyan.*

THE AUTHOR'S EXPERIENCE IN THE TREATMENT OF DISEASES.

The fact being established that disease is either a local or general impediment to the nerve force that rules the human machine, then all disease can be grouped under the headings "local" and "general" nervous diseases.

Trusting that my experience in such diseases may aid the medical profession and laity in preventing or allaying them, I give my experience in a few words:

I am of the opinion that a large percentage of the medical profession, when called upon to diagnose and treat nerve cases, do not lay stress enough upon the condition of the patient's mind, failing to realize fully that the mind, dwelling at the head of the nervous system, governs the amount of nerve force generated in and radiated from the brain. I believe, further, that the medical profession, generally, fails to consider sufficiently the effect of abnormal thought upon the physical; that perhaps the experience of many physicians with purely nervous diseases has been somewhat limited and that they have not profited by their experiences with such diseases, or have failed entirely to diagnose and treat them as such.

Let us review some of our frequent sayings: The nervous system is to the physical, what the foundation is to the building. If in any manner the foundation is weakened, the structure begins to topple; when the foundation is strengthened the structure is correspondingly strengthened.

The nervous system, to review its main features, consists of the brain (the dynamo) and the spinal cord, from which issue the 41 pairs of nerves and their infinite number of branches some of them so small as to be almost invisible, even under a high-power microscope.

The nervous system can well be compared with a hose-pipe system, even the minutest nerves being hollow to all intents and purposes, since their function is to convey brain fluid (nerve force) to all parts of the body to which they extend. Imagine the fine consistency of the brain fluid (nerve force) that permeates all the tissues of the body through these nerves. Have you sufficiently considered the duties imposed upon the brain as a dynamo, engine, power-house? Have you not again and again noted the effect upon the physical condition of the patient who has handicapped his brain by excessive mental work, grief, hurry, worry, hatred, envy, anger, jealousy, malice, resentment, mental depression, excesses or inharmonies of any sort?

There is enough nerve force generated in the brain under normal conditions, to supply the entire system with energy or strength. Do you think it possible for a normal, physical condition to be maintained when 50 per cent. or more of this nerve force or energy is dissipated in abnorman thought or otherwise? A normal circulation is dependent upon a normal nerve supply. When the transmission of nerve force is impeded, perversion of circulation is the effect. A healthy condition depends upon a normal circulation, and as the circulatory system is governed by the nervous system, the medical profession will all agree that when the brain (the dynamo) is handicapped in its generation and distribution of energy, a general perversion of circulation is the effect, hence a general diseased condition. The alimentary tract, heart, lungs, liver, kidneys, in fact, the entire system is robbed of blood as well as of nerve force upon which they are dependent for the performance of their functions.

It is the continued mental resistance of things real and imaginary that often eventually places one in a condition requiring treatment. Waste makes want in the human system as well as in one's finances. Waste of nerve force, due to abnormal thought or excesses, will eventually bankrupt the health. One's storehouse of nerve force or vitality should be guarded with as much consideration as a bank account. It is worry and waste, not work, that kills. The good floater who glides along with the current and keeps his head above water, survives longest, while he who "bucks the stream" is sure to go under.

Thoughts precede words and actions, determine to a large extent man's condition, and mold his future. which is conclusive evidence that mind is about all that counts in man.

Mind is to the brain and body as is the electrical engineer to the power-house and street-car system, or the engineer to the locomotive and train of cars. Notice here that "mind" is all this, rather than brain, which is often considered mind instead of its agent.

How many have been robbed of appetite by sorrow, worry, anger, hatred, depression, over-mental exertion, etc.! Every thought is recorded at the solar (sun) plexus from which radiates, apparently, all nerve force, but which is, in reality, generated in and radiated from the brain. The solar plexus is one of the many servants of the mind—it responds to every thought, be it good or bad. Every despondent or harrowing thought apparently closes or contracts this plexus, robbing it of nerve force and hindering its radiation of energy, while every happy or wholesome thought opens or relaxes the same, and stimulates or promotes its radiation of energy, thus producing harmony which is health, inharmony being disease.

Nerve patients (I call them "nerve" patients out of policy rather than nervous patients, it has a better effect upon them) frequently become depleted to the extent that they are susceptible to any disease, the cause, in the majority of cases I have treated being clearly a leakage of nerve force from an "open valve" or excesses, while the balance were attributable to mechanical pressure.

Our minds are not unlike our physical selves; after laboring during the day, we could not expect to rest and recuperate by working all night, but after laboring during the day, mental workers deplete their nervous systems by taking their business home with them to finish or worry about at night, when their minds should be relaxed and given a chance to recuperate.

SYMPTOMS IN NERVOUS DISEASES.

The symptoms in nerve depletion are: a general weakened condition, fatigue from slight exertion, indigestion, constipation, functional heart trouble, tired feeling at the base of brain, impaired vision, shallow breathing, frequent micturition (which causes the patient to suspect kidney disease), tendency to avoid conversation, forgetfulness, insomnia, horrible dreams and a contracted condition of the muscles and tissues of the entire body. Darting pains are liable to occur anywhere between the top of the head and the bottom of the feet. A strange mental condition frequently takes possession of the patient, causing him to fear that his mind will become unbalanced. The brain is not unlike any other part of the human system, the more it is exercised the more blood and nerve force are required to supply it.

Nerve patients, as a rule, endure so much mental suffering that they readily accept any treatment recommended, they are "grasping for straws." A patient, probably after having had all kinds of treatment and taken all kinds of medicine without benefit, is often finally advised by his physician to "take a trip to the mountains," when in reality what he needs most are the comforts of home and the ministrations of friends. He is nervous, and if questioned as to whether or not he is mentally disturbed, he will almost invariably say "no," but when told that the symptoms clearly indicate the fact that he is or has been, he will admit that "he has been worrying a little." He has tried to "cross bridges" before coming to them, and has anticipated fearful occurrences upon which he has never realized, except in loss of energy, and has carried real and imaginary burdens of his own and all his friends. In fact, his condition may all be caused by or summed up in the one word FEAR—always fearing something and cultivating a crop of mental weeds, thus dwarfing normal thought.

TREATMENT OF NERVOUS DISEASES.

The foregoing class, or for that matter, any other class of patients might be treated for a year, and if then asked the question: "In what way does your physician expect to restore your health, energy or vitality; has he diagnosed your case correctly by finding the CAUSE of the disease, if so, is he working on the CAUSE with the view of removing it that the effect (disease) may be removed?" The patient nine times out of ten could not answer intelligently. Therefore your consultation room should be provided with a skeleton and good anatomical charts, showing not only the nervous system, but the entire human system. Explain the nervous system; explain that the brain is at the head of it; explain what is required of the brain and how easily the nervous system can be depleted by abnormal thought, excesses, etc. and the results of such depletion. Show the patient how either structural defect or pressure produces disease. When you have charts and skeleton with which to explain that disease is a condition produced by either a mechanical or mental impediment to the nerve force that runs the human machine, you will almost invariably

secure prospective patients from the casual in-
quirers. They will learn more of the anatomy of
the human system in a five-minute explanation
than they would in the same number of months
without them, because they have a picture before
them with which to associate an explanation,
therefore, will retain it.

One cannot expect to give, in five or ten minutes,
an exhaustive explanation of how disease is produced in the human body, or one that can be retained in the mind clearly after the patient goes
home, therefore, you should always have on hand
for patients (prospective or otherwise) to take
home with them, the best written medium through
which they can acquire a knowledge of the mental
and mechanical causes of disease and the means
for their removal. Your patients will undoubtedly
be interested by the chart explanation and the literature you hand to them now will surely be read,
—it will be re-read another day—then most likely
it will be given by them to some one else having
similar symptoms, to explain his or her maladies.
So, these lucid explanations and good literature
are well worth your time for many reasons.

When treating nervous patients a large percentage of the physicians "when in doubt" as to
cause, have resorted to an experimental treatment. Do you, "when in doubt" as to cause, limit
your treatment to a stereotyped prescription or

process that will handicap nature instead of helping her? Do you, when arrogating unto yourself the name of "physician," realize that you are only a helper—that NATURE is the physician, ALWAYS HAS BEEN AND ALWAYS WILL BE, and that it is your duty, with the cooperation of the patient, to FIND AND REMOVE THE CAUSE, thus enabling NATURE to effect a cure? Should these patients receive a stereotyped treatment, when the knowledge or experience of the practitioner in the treatment of such conditions will not enable him to LOCATE THE EXACT CAUSE? I should say certainly not. YOU ARE NOT WORKING UPON NOR REMOVING THE CAUSE OF THE DISEASE. A cure depends largely upon a CORRECT DIAGNOSIS, but you have not made such—YOU HAVE NOT LOCATED THE CAUSE.

If my experience in the treatment of these average nervous diseases counts for anything, the majority has been caused, primarily, by abnormal mental exertion and excesses. The patients have been on the verge of a nervous collapse at time of treatment, or have suffered from nerve depletion in the past; the motor has been handicapped; there has been a leakage of nerve force—an "open valve," which acts on the same principle as a leakage from a bucket of water—a constant dripping will soon deplete the contents of the bucket.

When treating these cases the majority of the medical profession has absolutely disregarded the foundation, the mind, where cause exists. Now is the time you may fail to secure satisfactory results, if you ever do, and you begin to doubt the virtue of your chosen profession; you now look to vibrators, batteries, baths, etc. in a blind endeavor to relieve the patient, but to no avail. While you have been looking for a leakage in the nervous system, due to structural defects or otherwise, you have over-looked the condition of the foundation, or rather that which is at the head of and governs the nervous system, the mind, the medium through which God supplies the patient with energy. The waste of energy must be stopped and manipulation or experimental treatment will not do it. You might treat the patient for six months in a harmless way, allowing NATURE to make partial repairs, but unless given the best advice as to the elimination of depleting thoughts, that have taken possession of his mind, he is liable at any time during an hour's mental depression, to set aside the benefits derived from your six months' treatment.

I am not decrying manipulation in these conditions. It is absolutely necessary to help restore a normal nerve and blood supply to the tissues that have been robbed. I do not claim that there has been an absence of apparent malposition of vertebrae in some of these cases, there probably has been, but I have cured my patients and at the same time been unable to reduce some apparent deviations. I have also been unable to "line up" the spine in such phenomenal time as has been stated in some of our case reports.

SECRET OF SUCCESS IN MENTAL MEDICINE.

The secret of success in mental medicine is to advise the patient so that by his cooperation his mind will be strengthened thus enabling him to eliminate the depleting thought which has taken possession of his mind. Show him that there is absence of nerve force and energy; that he is depleted physically and must regain strength. Teach him that he must acquire nerve force and conserve the same by keeping the "valves" closed, that is, avoiding excitement, anger, hatred, depressions, excessive mental and physical exertion, etc. Advise patients to be calm at all times, that the mental condition of fear must be set aside; that depressing thought is their worst enemy. If one declines positively to entertain a thought it will "take wings" almost immediately—allow it to take possession of the mind, it will be most difficult to banish.

Teach patients to reason with their thoughts as they would with members of their family—that thoughts are things. Explain to them that there is absolutely nothing which they should fear, pre-

vail upon them to forget the past, to live in the
present and not to "cross bridges" before coming
to them. Explain to them that the physical is
suffering from want of nerve force due to an
"open valve" in the dynamo, and that in order to
restore health the leakage must be stopped—that
a leakage of nerve force is like a leakage of water
from a bucket—that the leakage must be stopped
by eliminating the depleting thought, and that in
order to do this, cooperation is necessary. Encourage your patient and explain to him that the
human system will be in a depleted condition just
as long as he wastes 50 per cent. or more of the
nerve force that is intended to maintain the same
in a healthy condition. If the patient persists in
entertaining the abnormal thought, after having
had its effect upon the nervous system explained
to him, the only recourse is to arouse his fear by
convincing him that a continuance in this line of
thought will result in either apoplexy, paralysis
or insanity; he will then be more apt to exert himself to eliminate the thought.

The patient's mind should be treated in a manner similar to that by which the farmer tills the
soil—uproot the weeds, that vegetation may
flourish!

The foregoing experience in the treatment of
nervous diseases may be a benefit to both the
medical profession and laity. Medical science

must be strengthened principally with the help of field members who have had practical experience in the treatment of disease, and who have given certain classes of disease special attention and study. One may remain in the clinic or recitation room for years, preparing to combat disease in the human system, but the student soon learns, when he enters the field of active practice, that his qualifications are very meager indeed, that the theories acquired so conscientiously and laboriously, frequently fail to fill the bill, that practical knowledge is necessary, and that suggestions from experienced members are most helpful. Case reports from the experiences of field members are requested to advance science and strengthen its foundation principles. How is medical science to be advanced if the profession, or a large percentage of it, insists that all its members entertain the same ideas as to the causation of disease? Advancement depends upon diversity of opinion, and if opinions founded upon years of experience are expressed at variance with those heretofore held, and tend to broaden the field of medical science, it is just and proper that they receive due consideration.

I have treated nearly 650 patients since June, 1900, approximately 500 of these were nerve cases; I failed to effect cures of possibly 10 per cent., but rarely ever failed to benefit, to some extent, the conditions of even these extreme cases. Every case of paralysis was preceded by nervous prostration which was the result of continued abnormal thought or excesses.

About 150 cases were due to structural defect, the predominating cause being a deviation of one of the innominates (hip-bones); other cases included tic-douloureux, facial neuralgia, gout, rheumatic conditions, etc., where loss of nerve force was due to intense pain, incident to pressure.

Would it not be well to broaden out a little and consider the experiences and suggestions of field members in regard to the causes and treatment of some diseases, as well as the causes to which the weaknesses of medical science are attributable? The public is quick to condemn and slow to investigate; such has also been the case with the different therapies (the different methods of treating disease). By reviewing the past we will see that wherever a progressive thought has been advanced in any age, ignorance, selfishness or prejudice has been ready to denounce it and to persecute the one who advanced it. Suggestions which tend toward the betterment of science should be given due attention. As yet, no one therapy has proved to be infallible and supreme.

A therapy should be adopted, based upon the principles of CAUSE AND EFFECT. Look to the nervous system, principally, for mental and mechanical causes, since the nerve force or energy generated in the brain and distributed to all parts of the body through the nerves can be impeded in only two ways—mechanically or mentally.

As the stability of a structure or science depends principally upon its foundation, and practitioners fail to recognize this great principle, they are limiting the foundation of medical science to structural defect, germ theories, diagnosing by taking pulse and temperature and noting condition of the tongue, thus ignoring the keystone in the arch forming the main dependence—state of mind.

To disregard the mental condition in the causation of disease is about as reasonable as to decry the hot foot bath and hot drinks when circulation is unequalized by a severe cold, "grip" etc., claiming that manipulation or drugs are all that is helpful or necessary. Would you necessarily look for a mechanical cause or germ in case of la-grippe or in diseased conditions due to severe colds?

PHYSICIAN PORTRAYED AS THE ENGINEER.

I have read articles by members of the medical profession in which they portrayed the physician as the engineer of the human system, at the same time attributing all diseased conditions to structural defects or germs.

219

If you considered yourself proficient as an engineer, and were running a steam engine, would you look for other than a lack of energy if the engine were laboring with difficulty to haul a train on 50 per cent. of the steam necessary to do it?

Would you look amongst wheels and machinery for cause or structural defects, or for other causes, if the engine failed to run a plant when 50 per cent. of a full head of steam was escaping from an open valve?

Should we, as physicians, feel justified in employing an engineer (?) who disregards the condition of the dynamo, motor or engine that generates the force necessary to run the machinery?

When called upon as an engineer to adjust the "human machine," are you, when diagnosing your cases, going to continue to limit your diagnosis to looking for structural defects, hunting for germs, taking of pulse and temperature and noting condition of tongue?

Would it not be wisdom to consider whether or not the cause is attributable to a defective dynamo or engine, which I have used in this discussion as a figure of speech for the mind, not the animal organism?

Do you not think it high time that the profession "wakes up" to realize the fact that there are potent causes for disease in the human system, other than mechanical, and that life, especially modern life, can not be run adequately on 50 per cent. of the energy or nerve force necessary? In asking this I mean to emphasize the necessity of doing more than to admit this truth as a matter of observation and reason—the necessity of making a place for it constantly in diagnosis and treatment. All know this contention to be true. None ever has disputed it, for it is axiomated. Yet few members of the medical profession actually make use of the fact, dividing his practice into the classes of "structural cause" and "mental cause" patients.

There is no intention to decry the medical profession, nor the efforts of any of its members, but to awaken it to a proper realization of the fact that there are more important features to be considered than structural defect and germ theories when diagnosing. The mind is a factor always present for weal or woe, and can seldom be overlooked with impunity.

Experience leads me to believe that there are TWO KINDS OF PRIMARY CAUSES necessary to produce disease in the human system, MENTAL or MECHANICAL. Practice convinces me than MIND WASTE, rather than "mechanical causes," is largely in the majority.

The Author's Astigmatic Chart, page 192, is 10x
20 inches, folds in center and has complete directions for use on back, also test-type attachment.
For sale by the author, 161 State St., Chicago, Ill.
Price 50 cents post-paid.

Printed in the USA
CPSIA information can be obtained
at www.ICGtesting.com
LVHW021112281223
767380LV00077B/106